eat
according to your
body type

eat
according to your
body type

150 AYURVEDIC VEGETARIAN RECIPES TO RESTORE YOUR HEALTH

DR LAKSHMI LAKSHMANAN

First published in India by HarperCollins *Publishers* 2025
HarperCollins *Publishers* India, Cyber City,
Building 10-A, Gurugram, Haryana – 122002, India
www.harpercollins.co.in

and
Indus Source
42/43C, Balaji Bhavan, Sakal Bhavan Road, Sector 11, CBD Belapur, Navi Mumbai 400614

Text excluding recipes © Dr Lakshmi Lakshmanan 2025
Recipes © Nirmala Lakshmanan 2025
Photographs © Shubham Jain 2025

10 9 8 7 6 5 4 3 2 1

P-ISBN: 978-93-7307-533-4
E-ISBN: 978-93-7307-435-1

The views and opinions expressed in this book are the author's own and the facts are as reported by her, and the publishers are not in any way liable for the same.
None of the content in this book is intended to be a substitute for professional medical advice and should not be relied on as health or medical advice, diagnosis or treatment. Always seek the guidance of your doctor or other qualified health professionals with any questions you may have regarding your health or a medical condition. The recipes in this book have been tested by the author to the best of her knowledge. Every effort has been made to verify the accuracy of the recipes contained herein, however, neither HarperCollins nor the author shall be held responsible for the outcome of any of the recipes. Individuals with allergies, special food requirements or health issues should determine the use or substitution of these recipes at their own risk. The appropriate nutrient values and allergen potential of each food source may vary for each individual. The information provided via the book is intended to be used as a guide only. HarperCollins and the author specifically disclaim all liability for the use of the recipes by the readers. Please consult your physician before making changes to your regular diet, or treatment.

Dr Lakshmi Lakshmanan asserts the moral right to be identified as the author of this work.

All rights reserved. No part of this publication may be reproduced, stored in a retrieval system, or transmitted, in any form or by any means, electronic, mechanical, photocopying, recording or otherwise, without the prior permission of the publishers.

Without limiting the exclusive rights of any author, contributor or the publisher of this publication, any unauthorized use of this publication to train generative artificial intelligence (AI) technologies is expressly prohibited. HarperCollins also exercise their rights under Article 4(3) of the Digital Single Market Directive 2019/790 and expressly reserve this publication from the text and data-mining exception.

Typeset in 11/14 Adobe Garamond Pro
by HarperCollins *Publishers* India Pvt. Ltd

Printed and bound at
Replika Press Pvt. Ltd.

This book is produced from independently certified FSC® paper to ensure responsible forest management.

*

HarperCollins *Publishers*, Macken House, 39/40 Mayor Street Upper, Dublin 1, D01 C9W8, Ireland

*To the three incredible women who have profoundly influenced
my life:*

*My beloved grandmother, Mrs Muthayee Palaniappan, who watches
over me from above;
My wonderful mother, Mrs Nirmala Lakshmanan, who has unwavering
faith in me;
and
My beautiful daughter, Ms Santhini Anoop, who motivates me every day.*

The detailed notes pertaining to this book are available on the HarperCollins website. Scan this QR code to access the same.

Contents

	Introduction	ix
1.	The Three Supporting Pillars of Life	1
2.	Nutrition According to Ayurveda	8
3.	Understanding Agni and Ama	17
4.	Shadrasa: The Six Tastes	20
5.	Prakriti: Your Constitution	25
6.	Eat for Your Mind	39
7.	Eat According to the Season and the Time of the Day	43
8.	Ten Rules to Eat Healthier	48
9.	Foundational Ayurvedic Foods and How to Prepare Them	50
10.	Cooking Pre-Prep	68
11.	Recipes for Vata	71
12.	Recipes for Pitta	135
13.	Recipes for Kapha	191
	Acknowledgements	247
	Notes	249

INTRODUCTION

'No one is born a great cook; one learns by doing.'
—Julia Child

I was not a fan of cooking during my adolescent years. My mom was a great cook, and she used to prepare tasty yet healthy recipes for me, even using ingredients I did not like but were needed to support my nutrition. She made a variety of foods ranging from beetroot pesto to hibiscus squash—innovations that I truly came to appreciate when I left home for college, where I missed her delicious cooking. The meals at the hostel mess were okay but could not compare to my mom's homemade dishes. Later, when I joined my first job and had to stay alone was when my cooking journey began. I never liked street food or eating from restaurants, definitely not on an everyday basis. So, I started cooking for myself. Initially, I found it difficult and time consuming. However, as time passed, I started enjoying the process and began trying new recipes, using the ideas that I read in the Ayurveda Samhitas (the classical textbooks of Ayurveda). During this phase of experimenting, I came to understand three things that I would like to share with you.

- Cooking is an essential life skill that encourages creativity and makes you feel good since it is a way to nurture yourself as well as others. It is good to start cooking at an early age. If possible, involve your children in the cooking process early so they start enjoying it as they grow up. My daughter and I cook together—it's fun and time well spent together, with the added benefit of minimizing her gadget use.

INTRODUCTION

Most kids have a lot of energy, and they love learning and doing new things. They are curious to know where food comes from and how it is prepared, so they tend to enjoy the process of cooking.

- Cooking at home gives you more control over the ingredients you put into your body. It also brings joy and contributes to good health. You can choose good-quality ingredients and cook fresh food, which is healthier than eating out.
- Cooking is an amazing exercise for your brain. The hands-on experience during cooking engages the five senses—sight, touch, smell, sound and taste. This helps to improve your sensory stimulation. When food looks nice, smells good and tastes yummy it satisfies all your senses and brings a sense of fulfilment.

Here I am now—a skilled Ayurveda nutrition counsellor and chef instructor. I love to cook and to teach. I have conducted Ayurvedic cooking workshops across India and abroad, and through these experiences I have gained insights into the relationship between health and food, which I have distilled into the recipes in this book.

Many people think that because Ayurveda originated in India, its rules can be applied only to Indian cuisine. However, this isn't true—the principles of Ayurveda are universal and can be applied everywhere, in any country and at any point in time. I present to you this cookbook to help you get started. This is a compilation of my most foolproof vegetarian recipes for good health, with simple instructions and preparation methods.

This Ayurveda recipe book is the outcome of years of continuous effort. I have been hosting Ayurveda-based holistic consultations and conferences on healthy living for more than fifteen years, and during these years what I understood was that people are motivated to change their diet to improve their health, but they face barriers of many sorts such as diet confusion, lack of time and feeling overwhelmed by the task. They finally end up rushing the process of cooking, which makes them unhappy and the outcome undesirable. If you are new to cooking, I want you to first understand that cooking is not as complicated as you think. If you are willing to learn, cooking can be simple and fun. You may have a love-hate relationship with cooking in the beginning but slowly, over a period of time, you will start to love it.

'The food you eat can be either the safest and most powerful form of medicine, or the slowest form of poison.'

—Ann Wigmore

Diet has a profound effect on the human body. Eating a healthy diet alone is not enough. What, when and how we eat are important as these factors affect our body and mind. For example, eating a healthy diet may not be nutritious if eaten at the wrong time, say at midnight, as our body needs time to digest before sleeping. Or eating a healthy diet but mixing incompatible foods (for example, having a hot meal with a cold juice) may produce adverse effects instead.

Today, most of us are conscious and curious about diet and nutrition and we tend to blindly follow information we get from the media. Sometimes, after following a specific diet pattern for many days, even months, we start thinking, 'Oh, I am not getting my desired result,' at which point we may visit a nutritionist or get online evaluations about a diet that we think is good for us. However, what we first need to realize is that not all types of food are suitable for everyone because we all have different body types and health needs. *One size does not fit all.* Information about diets is widely available; thus, it is general and not specific. Ayurveda, on the other hand, offers customized nutrition advice and explains the suitability of a particular diet for people with specific constitutions to achieve good health. We know that diet is considered the 'greater medicine', but it should be tailored according to our constitution to get our desired results. A diet that is suitable for you may not be suitable for someone else. For example, natural sweets are good for people who wish to gain weight (Vata body type), but they might not be okay for people suffering from metabolic problems like obesity and diabetes (Kapha body type).

Your diet is the basis of life, strength, growth, development, immunity, etc. Food nourishes your body; you cannot sustain life without a proper diet. When there is harmony of the body and mind, you desire healthy food and vice versa. This is because the body and mind are interconnected and influence your food choices. You crave chocolates or candies when you are stressed. A person suffering from anaemia may have a greater inclination towards eating ice or raw rice. When your body–mind harmony is out of balance, you make mistakes in choosing the right foods.

Diet is explored in detail in Ayurveda. According to its principles, you should follow a diet that is opposite in nature to your prakriti (your unique body type). 'Like attracts like'—that is a diet that enhances a dosha (your constitution) and can aggravate it, leading to an imbalance. On the other hand, a diet that reduces the dosha's intensity will soothe it. For example, if you have too much dryness in the body (dry skin, dry and rough hair, dryness in the intestine causing a tendency towards constipation), include a good amount of ghee or oil in each meal. If you have sluggish lymphatic circulation and a tendency towards water retention in the body, then reduce the intake of juicy vegetables and fruits. That is why it is important to know your prakriti and choose an appropriate diet to live a healthy, disease-free life.

In this book, I have incorporated Ayurvedic principles to create recipes for the different prakritis. These recipes can be prepared quickly and with minimal fuss, so even if you are a busy person you may be able to find time to prepare fresh, delicious meals. I encourage you to try the recipes and to feel relaxed and try again if you do not get it right the first time. Not all are born great cooks, but you can become one. Remember, practice makes perfect.

1
THE THREE SUPPORTING PILLARS OF LIFE

'If we could give every individual the right amount of nourishment and exercise, not too little and not too much, we would have found the safest way to health.'

—Hippocrates

TRAYOPASTHAMBHA

Just like the pillars of a building provide support to the structure, trayopasthambha or the 'three supporting pillars of life'—proper diet (ahara), good sleep (nidra) and a moral code of life (brahmacharya)—support our body structure and functions.

According to Ayurveda, these three basic tools are important to maintain good health and protect our body from diseases. If we are negligent of these three pillars, which is the case with most people today, it leads to an increased risk of disease and decreases one's longevity.

1. **Ahara**: Food is the source of life. The growth and development of our body and mind depend upon the nature of our diet. Food not only provides us with physical nutrition, it also governs our sensorial, mental and spiritual well-being. The therapeutic properties of an Ayurveda diet are largely defined by the energy of taste or rasa. Ayurveda explains the different ways of preparing food that are aimed at altering certain properties, or as an antidote

to the possible side effects of the food itself. Today, fast food is focused only on taste, so we become addicted to it without considering its nutritional quality. Ayurveda says that food should be prepared keeping in mind the effect it will have on the health of our body and mind. It lays down certain codes of conduct for eating that are important for good health. These are as follows:

- Eat in pleasant and quiet surroundings; sit in one place and eat.
- Focus on the food while eating. Avoid eating in a hurry or too slowly, and refrain from speaking while eating.
- Consume food that is fresh, warm, tasty and easy to digest according to one's constitution, the season and the time.
- Eat only after the previous meal is digested.
- Eat food in a proper quantity.
- The food items in a meal should not contradict one another in their actions or compatibilities. For example, the consumption of milk and sour fruits together should be avoided.
- Eating a wide range of foods is good for our immunity, so one should include all the six tastes—sweet, sour, salty, pungent, bitter and astringent—in one's diet. But an excess of anything must be avoided.

The occasional consumption of unwholesome or incompatible food, or food not recommended for one's constitution, does not have a notable ill effect. Although it is always good to avoid foods that may aggravate the dominant dosha in our constitution, it is not always possible for us to do so because of socializing, or sometimes we fall prey to our temptations. It is okay to indulge occasionally but be careful not to have incompatible food on a regular basis and in high quantities as it can lead to the rapid formation of microtoxins, which accumulate in the cells and cause inflammation, ultimately disrupting the body's natural defence mechanisms.[1]

2. **Nidra**: Sleep is an essential need because our body recharges its energy stores through rest. Adults need at least seven to nine hours of sleep at night. Today, even children struggle to get enough sleep and most adults are getting no more than six hours of sleep due to work pressures and an unhealthy work–life balance.[2] Hence, people tend to sleep more on the weekends to help the body recover from the hours of sleep lost. But does it really help? The answer is no. This just messes up your internal clock (known as the circadian rhythm), which becomes out of sync with your environment. The adverse effect of untimely, inadequate or excessive sleep is immense.

We have more conveniences nowadays, like temperature regulation (air-conditioning for the summer and heating in the winter), comfortable beds and pillows, soothing music, etc., but these come at a cost. Distractions in the form of smartphones and TVs in the bedroom make us spend more time being awake instead of taking time to sleep. Sound sleep improves focus, memory, cognitive performance, sensory function, digestion, metabolism and overall health.[3] In this book, I will show you how you can reset your schedule to the right time, according to your body type as specified in Ayurvedic texts.

Are you getting enough sleep?

Read the questions and mark your answer in the relevant column. When you finish answering all the questions, count the total number of A's, B's, C's and D's you got to calculate your score.

Question	Rarely (A)	Occasionally (B)	Frequently (C)	Almost every day (D)
Do you wake up easily when the alarm goes off?				
Are you in a good mood during the day?				
Are you able to focus and remember things without difficulty?				
Do you feel physically energetic during the day?				
Is it easy to get through the day without caffeine?				
On average, do you get six to eight hours of sleep every night?				
Are you fast asleep when you are in bed?				

Your score:

If you have:

- More D's, then congratulations! You are getting more than enough sleep!
- More C's, then you have average sleep. It is okay, but you should aim for better sleep.
- More B's, then your sleep is not good. You are definitely pulling through the day. You should sleep more.
- More A's, then you have a serious case of sleep deprivation. You need to fix it immediately.

3. **Brahmacharya**: Sex plays a very crucial role in our lives. It is as important as food. Eating less food produces a state of malnutrition while excess intake leads to obesity. Similarly, less and unsatisfactory sex or compulsive sexual behaviour can cause distress and problems in one's relationship, health, job and other facets of life. Sexual energy is simply another form of creative energy. However, it is very concentrated and powerful, as any stimulation, be it visual (watching videos or images related to it), auditory (music or moaning sounds) or tactile (caress or kiss), can be highly arousing for many individuals. That is, it seems to gain its own momentum and urgency, making it difficult to get control over it. Mind control significantly diminishes the feeling that sexual fulfilment is the sole means of dealing with the intense sexual reaction. It helps you think and understand (visceral and not intellectual understanding) how energy moves through your body and how you can divert this energy to any place you want. This makes you conscious of the trigger factors. As sexual arousal is not only a physiological response and is influenced by cognitive processes, you can always shift your focus away from the strong stimuli that initiate the arousal. Techniques like mindfulness and meditation, which involve focusing on the

present moment without judgment, can also help in managing arousal by increasing awareness of thoughts and feelings without getting carried away by them.

Sigmund Freud's psychoanalytic theory explains that a person can redirect their base desires or instincts into socially acceptable and higher pursuits. This redirection of energy helps in healthy psychological functioning and contributes to cultural development. According to him, human personality has three parts: 'id—the primitive desires', 'ego—the reality-oriented self' and 'superego—the moral conscience'. The ego uses defence mechanisms to find ways to cope with conflicts arising from the id's demands and the superego's restrictions and realities of the external world. Sublimation is one such defence mechanism where the ego redirects strong desires or impulses into other constructive activities. So when intense sexual desire arises, that energy might be channelled into artistic creativity or competitive sports, for instance.[4] We should pay attention to our body and emotions before and during sex so as to be aware and mindful and to accept our sexuality. In yogic tradition, improper use of sexual energy is considered to be the greatest obstacle to spiritual enlightenment. The thought of sex provokes the mind. Hence, controlled/healthy thoughts regarding sex are more important.

Sexual energy is a life force that exists in all of us. It is inextricably linked not only to our sexual drives and desires, but also to our connectedness to others. Balanced sexual behaviour is key to a happy and healthy life. Sexual discipline is a required trait in today's world— one should satisfy their sexual desires in a civilized manner rather than a destructive one. Each individual possesses a unique sexual identity. Our thoughts, feelings, desires and perspectives on sex are shaped by our cultural background and personal experiences, yet they primarily reflect our dosha. Gaining insight into our dosha and its impact on our sexuality can enrich the significance of sex in our lives and relationships. Additionally, understanding our partner's dosha is crucial, as it enables us to fulfil their needs, informs our approach to intimacy, and fosters patience and empathy when our sexual experiences do not meet our expectations.

- Vata body types have an erratic interest in sex. They have low energy levels and may get easily exhausted by frequent sex.
- Pitta-predominant persons are passionate and have a strong desire for sex, but they can experience burn-out if they're not mindful about their sexual indulgences.
- Kapha constitution people have the most sexual vitality. They have a constant but moderate interest in sex and good stamina.

If you harness the power of your sexual energy correctly, it can help you achieve greater success in all areas of your life and lead to a more fulfilling existence. Channelling sexual desire into higher pursuits is possible only by taming the mind.

2
NUTRITION ACCORDING TO AYURVEDA

'Good nutrition creates health in all areas of our existence. All parts are interconnected.'

—Dr T. Colin Campbell

Today, it is easier to eat an unhealthy diet, with modern lifestyles seeing an increased consumption of high-energy food, unhealthy fats, sugar and salt. A nutritious diet helps to maintain proper digestion and metabolism, supports normal growth and development, strengthens the immune system, nourishes the body and reduces the risk of chronic diseases, thus contributing to overall health. Inadequate nutrition leads to the depletion of energy, body mass, procreative ability, weakening of immunity, shortening of lifespan and disturbed functioning of mental faculties, intellect and senses. Malnutrition leads to health problems like anaemia, vitamin B12 deficiency, folate deficiency, etc. However, overnutrition leads to fatigue, weakness, lethargy, weight gain, impaired digestion, sleep issues, etc., and it increases the risk of lifestyle-related metabolic problems such as diabetes, hypertension, cardiovascular diseases and obesity.[5]

Nutritional intervention helps to prevent and reverse lifestyle disorders. You can hardly influence the air you breathe in. But diet can be influenced as it is totally up to you to choose what you eat and drink. Ayurveda offers a lot of freedom to choose the right food for you.

UNDERSTANDING AHARA

> *'What most people don't realize is that food is not just calories: It's information. It actually contains messages that communicate to every cell in the body.'*
>
> —Dr Mark Hyman

'Ahara' constitutes anything we take in—including food, water, breath, emotions and information through our sense organs. Nutrition refers to the supply of essential materials in the form of food and oxygen to cells and organisms, which is vital for sustaining life. Adequate nutrition also helps to prevent common health problems and repair damaged tissues.

The food components that we consume can be classified into four varieties:

1. **Aashit:** Soft food like cooked rice, cooked vegetables such as carrots, sweet potatoes and zucchini, and fruits like bananas, ripe mangoes, etc.
2. **Peeta:** Fluids like milk, water, etc.
3. **Leeda:** Semi-solid foods like khichadi, cooked lentils, etc.
4. **Khadit:** Coarse foods like salads and nuts

Ayurveda has listed twelve food groups with different nutritional values that are explained in the table below:

Food group in Sanskrit	Food group in English	Nutritional value
Shookadhanya	Cereals	Rich source of carbohydrates
Shamidhanya	Pulses	Rich in protein
Mamsa Varga	Meat	Good source of protein, minerals and fats

Food group in Sanskrit	Food group in English	Nutritional value
Shaaka Varga	Green leafy vegetables	Rich in roughage, antioxidants, vitamins and minerals
Phala Varga	Fruits	Rich in carbohydrates, antioxidants, vitamins, minerals and electrolytes
Harita Varga	Salads	Rich in roughage, vitamins and minerals
Madhya Varga	Fermented preparations	Rich in antioxidants and carbohydrates
Ambu Varga	Water	Hydrates the body, is rich in minerals and is an elixir
Gorasa Varga	Milk and its products	Rich in fats, proteins and carbohydrates
Ikshu Varga	Sugarcane and its products	A source of carbohydrates
Kritanna Varga	Pre-processed or ready-to-eat food like pickles, condiments (pesto), papad (roasted lentil crisps), etc.	Good source of functional components such as proteins, vitamins, minerals and phytochemicals
Aharayoni Varga	Food adjuvants like salt, oil and pepper	Improves taste and aroma and is a rich source of antioxidants

There is no better medicine than food. You will not succumb to disease if you consume the appropriate foods in the right quantities. Complexion, clarity, a good voice, a long life, understanding, happiness, satisfaction, growth, strength and intelligence are all achieved through proper nutrition. Food not only nourishes the body but also the mind.

EAT ACCORDING TO YOUR BODY TYPE

Whatever is beneficial for worldly happiness and spiritual salvation is said to be established through food.

Listening to your body

However, eating healthy food alone is not enough. One can derive ideal nutrition from a diet that is qualitatively and quantitatively balanced. Below are some signs that indicate you have consumed the right quantity of food:

- Feeling satisfied after a meal
- Not feeling heavy or sleepy
- Able to resume work easily without discomfort
- Active sense organs and mind
- Feeling of light appetite after approximately three to four hours

Your Ayurveda physician or nutritionist can guide you based on your prakriti, the state of your agni, health problems, the season, etc., but the first step is to *listen to your body*. You are the only person who knows the needs of your body so you must be conscious of the changes happening in your body and mind. For example, you may feel less hungry when you are resting more, while you may feel the need to eat more when you have to work longer hours than usual. If you do a physically laborious job, you might have the desire to eat more, whereas if you do a mentally demanding job, you might not need more food but what you may need is good exercise to balance mental stress.

IMMUNITY

'The natural healing force within each of us is the greatest force in getting well.'

—Hippocrates

'Ojas' is the vitality of the human body that sustains health and youthfulness. This is a unique concept in Ayurveda, which can be considered akin to immunity. Healthy food, proper digestion and a well-functioning metabolism nourish ojas and help maintain its balance. The quality of ojas depends on the health of body tissues and the equilibrium of the doshas.

Ojas can be described as the essence of all bodily tissues and an indicator of overall strength. If you closely look at ojas, its attributes are similar to those of Kapha dosha. Therefore, foods that nourish Kapha dosha also contribute to the maintenance of ojas. From the moment we are in our mother's womb, her diet and lifestyle begin shaping our ojas. However, later in life, we can enhance it through a balanced diet, regular exercise and sufficient rest. Ojas is deeply connected to the heart, mind, sense organs and body tissues. It is the body's natural elixir providing vigour, vitality, strength, radiance, immunity, energy and liveliness. At the emotional and spiritual level, it is the expression of one's consciousness.

When ojas is weakened, our immunity is compromised. Therefore, it is essential to follow a healthy diet as per Ayurvedic principles to preserve and nourish it.

NUTRITIONAL ERRORS

'Some things you have to do every day. Eating seven apples on Saturday night instead of one a day just isn't going to get the job done.'

—Jim Rohn

Sometimes, despite eating a healthy diet, you might still make a few nutritional errors—such as choosing inappropriate foods, developing unhealthy eating habits, combining incompatible foods, or eating at irregular times. Often, this happens simply due to a lack of awareness. Ayurveda recognizes the importance of these nutritional errors in contributing to diseases, categorizing them under the term 'Nindita Ashana' (unwholesome eating). Understanding these errors is essential so you can avoid them and make better food choices.

Here are some nutritional errors according to Ayurveda:

- **Anashana** (Consuming no food or complete fasting): Different fasting techniques—such as intermittent fasting—may not suit all body types. While fasting is often promoted as a detoxification method, Ayurveda suggests that rather than completely avoiding food, it is better to consume light, easily digestible foods like soups or fruits.
- **Pramitashana** (Habitual intake of food in extremely small quantities): Unless you are on complete rest, eating too little can deprive the body of the energy it needs to function. Historically, sanyasis (spiritual ascetics) survived on minimal food, as they spent most of their lives meditating in forests or mountains. However, modern-day sanyasis often engage in social activism or even political life in cities, requiring a different dietary approach. For everyone, consuming an adequate quantity of food is essential to support cellular functions and overall well-being.
- **Mahashana** (Overeating): More often than not, your meals are accompanied by distractions—reading, watching TV, scrolling through your phone, or discussing work. When your mind is elsewhere, you tend to eat more than what your body actually needs. Ayurveda views food as sacred, and eating while distracted is not only disrespectful to the meal but also harmful for digestion. Overeating can strain the digestive system, leading to digestive issues, weight gain and metabolic disorders. Mindful eating is key to preventing this.
- **Ajirnashana** (Consuming food during indigestion): Sometimes, social situations—such as office parties or family gatherings—lead you to eat despite having indigestion. Or perhaps when someone offers you your favourite sweet, you simply can't resist. However, eating when

digestion is already compromised only worsens the issue, overloading your system and delaying recovery. Frequent overeating, incompatible food combinations and irregular eating habits all contribute to indigestion. If digestion is already impaired, eating again before your body has fully processed the previous meal can lead to further complications.

- **Viruddhashana** (Consuming incompatible food): With busy schedules, many people only manage two or three meals a day, often loading their plates with a variety of foods without considering whether the combinations are beneficial or harmful. For example, a typical breakfast might include a cup of coffee, toast with butter or cheese, yoghurt and a glass of orange juice. While vitamin C from citrus fruits is excellent for immunity, combining it with dairy (such as milk tea or coffee) can create digestive issues. This is a classic example of an incompatible food combination that many people consume unknowingly. I've explained more about these combinations in Chapter 10.

- **Vishamashana** (Irregular eating habits or eating without following a specific time): One of the most common dietary mistakes is not eating at regular times. In today's fast-paced world, many people struggle to maintain consistent mealtimes. Late dinners are especially common because families often wait for everyone to finish work before eating together. Sales and marketing professionals, who travel frequently, often grab snacks on the go. Night-shift workers may eat at odd hours to stay awake. All of these habits disrupt digestion and overall health. Ayurveda emphasizes the importance of eating at fixed times to maintain digestive balance.

- **Adhyashana** (Eating again within a short time after a meal or eating before the previous meal is digested): Eating before the previous meal has been properly digested is a key factor in health problems like insulin resistance, sluggish metabolism and obesity. A full meal takes at least three to four hours to digest, so eating soon after can overload your system. Many people experience this issue at work, where meal breaks are fixed. Even if you're still full from your previous meal, you

may eat anyway to avoid feeling hungry later. Over time, this can impair digestion and metabolic function.
- **Samashana** (Consuming suitable and unsuitable foods): Understanding your prakriti is crucial for selecting the right diet. For instance, Kapha body types already have abundant moisture and oiliness in their systems, so consuming excessive juicy vegetables or oily foods may aggravate their natural tendencies.

Most of these nutritional errors can be avoided if you eat consciously. Ayurveda teaches us that food is not just fuel, it is a powerful tool for maintaining health and balance. By paying attention to what, when and how you eat, you can support your body's natural rhythms and improve your overall well-being.

Eating with Awareness: More than Just Personal Preference

Many people choose food based on personal cravings, body image goals or emotional comfort. But Ayurveda teaches us that food is primarily a source of prana—vital energy—that sustains life, and our intake should reflect this.

While modern nutrition focuses on caloric value and macronutrient distribution, Ayurveda emphasizes the taste, properties and digestive impact of food, as well as how your body processes it. From an Ayurvedic perspective, digestion is more important than simply counting calories. After all, what's the point of prescribing a 1,200-calorie diet if your body struggles to digest or assimilate it?

This doesn't mean Ayurveda disregards dietary requirements. In fact, it provides specific nutritional guidelines based on age, sex, season, geography, occupation and health conditions. For example, young individuals in a growth phase require heavier, more nourishing foods, whereas older adults benefit from lighter, antioxidant-rich meals.

Ayurvedic texts also outline dietary recommendations for pregnancy, providing a month-by-month diet plan to support both mother and baby. Similarly, Ayurveda classifies foods based on their effects in different conditions. For instance:

- Rice and sugar enhance lactation.
- Black gram supports spermatogenesis.
- Green leafy vegetables help relieve constipation.

Nutrition for healthy individuals and those recovering from illness is categorized as:

- **Hita Ahara:** A wholesome, health-promoting diet
- **Ahita Ahara:** An unhealthy, imbalanced diet
- **Pathya Ahara:** Foods that support recovery and well-being
- **Apathya Ahara:** Foods that are harmful or aggravate imbalances

3

UNDERSTANDING AGNI AND AMA

'All disease begins in the gut.'

—Hippocrates

Agni simply means 'fire', which is one of the five elements of the universe. In Ayurveda, agni represents the fire element within the body.

Fire is fast; it gives heat and light. Most importantly, fire is a powerful force of transformation. The sun, the ultimate source of energy—a concentrated ball of fire—is the largest form of agni in the universe. All natural processes on earth are directly or indirectly connected to the sun. For example, plants convert sunlight into chemical energy through photosynthesis.

Fire also has the power to transform raw food into cooked food. In the same way, agni converts ingested food into energy, which is responsible for all our vital bodily functions. For food to sustain and nourish life, it must be digested, absorbed and assimilated—a process governed by agni in our digestive system. In this way, agni fuels our growth, nourishment, strength, complexion, lustre, immunity, energy and overall vitality. A well-functioning agni is key to living a happy, healthy and long life.

Agni generates biological energy within each and every cell in our body. However, its main seat is the duodenum. This is because nutrients enter the stomach first, where they are subjected to the action of digestive fire. The digestive fire then transforms this food so that the metabolic fire can utilize it. The agni within our gastrointestinal tract is known as jataragni (digestive fire), while the agni present in our body's cells is called dhatvagni (metabolic fire).

AGNI AND GUT HEALTH

Your digestive tract is home to 95 per cent of your body's microflora. These gut microbes provide essential health benefits, particularly in regulating immune homeostasis. Your microbiome plays a crucial role in digestion, metabolism and overall development.[6] The good bacteria in your gut help break down food and protect you by crowding out harmful pathogens while also strengthening your immune system.

However, digestive problems arise when this balance is disrupted, allowing the bad bacteria to flourish. To maintain gut health, you need to support a balanced intestinal ecology by following a diet suited to your prakriti.

The Role of Agni in Nutrition and Health

Your overall nutrition depends on the proper functioning of agni and the regular excretion of waste from your body. To support agni, you should eat mindfully—without distractions such as televisions, mobile phones, books, or work discussions. This allows you to recognize when your stomach is three-quarters full and to stop eating when it is so, helping to prevent overeating or under-eating. Ayurveda views eating as a sadhana (a mindful practice), to be approached with focus and reverence. If eating is done absentmindedly, you may end up consuming too much or too little, disrupting your body's balance.

The Four States of Agni

Agni does not function the same way in everyone. It can be categorized into four states:

- **Sama Agni:** Balanced agni, which ensures good digestion and maintains the equilibrium of the doshas.

- **Vishama Agni**: Erratic agni, associated with excess Vata, leading to irregular metabolism, fluctuating appetite and unpredictable digestion.
- **Tikshna Agni**: Excessively strong agni, linked to excess Pitta, resulting in hypermetabolism and undernourishment.
- **Manda Agni**: Weak agni, caused by excess Kapha, leading to slow digestion, lethargy and excessive weight gain.

THE CONCEPT OF AMA: THE ROOT OF DISEASE

In everyday language, ama means immature, unripe, or undigested. In Ayurveda, it refers to toxic metabolic waste that accumulates when digestion is weak or incomplete.

Ama can be compared to endotoxins in the body or what modern medicine calls 'free radicals'. But it is a far more complex concept. Imagine the clogs that form in your kitchen sink or shower head—if properly maintained, blockages don't develop. Similarly, ama builds up in your body when your digestion is weak, creating a toxic sludge that disrupts cellular function.

If left unchecked, ama has the power to aggravate the doshas, disrupt homeostasis and initiate disease processes. In fact, most internal diseases begin with the formation of ama. Ayurveda teaches us that by keeping our agni strong and digestion optimal, we can prevent or slow down ama accumulation, thereby maintaining long-term health.

4
SHADRASA: THE SIX TASTES

'You have to taste a culture to understand it.'
— Deborah Cater

Taste is experienced when food comes into contact with the tongue. Your taste buds are capable of recognizing six distinct tastes, but most people have a natural preference for certain flavours and tend to overindulge in them. This can lead to imbalances, as a diet dominated by a single taste fails to provide complete nutrition.

To maintain good health, it is essential to include all six tastes in your daily diet.

The six tastes are explained in Ayurveda as Shadrasa ('shad' means 'six' and 'rasa' means 'taste'). They are as follows:

- **Madhura:** Sweet
- **Amla:** Sour
- **Lavana:** Salty
- **Tikta:** Bitter
- **Katu:** Pungent/Spicy
- **Kashaya:** Astringent

The table below illustrates the six tastes with examples, their elemental composition, their effect on the doshas and their properties:

Tastes	Mahabhuta Composition	Effect on Doshas	Properties	Examples
Sweet	Earth + Water	↑ Kapha ↓ Pitta ↓ Vata	Heavy, cold, unctuous	Milk, rice, wheat, sweet potatoes, carrots, beets
Sour	Earth + Fire	↑ Kapha ↑ Pitta ↓ Vata	Light, hot, unctuous	Sour fruits, lime, sour cream, vinegar, fermented food, cheese
Salty	Water + Fire	↑ Kapha ↑ Pitta ↓ Vata	Heavy, hot, unctuous	Rock salt, sea salt, gypsum salt, seaweed
Bitter	Air + Space	↑ Kapha ↓ Pitta ↓ Vata	Light, cold and dry	Black tea, dandelion root, myrrh, fenugreek, aloe, bitter leafy vegetables, bitter melon
Pungent	Fire + Air	↑ Kapha ↑ Pitta ↓ Vata	Light, hot, dry	Black pepper, ginger, jalapenos, garlic, cayenne pepper, wasabi
Astringent	Air + Earth	↑ Kapha ↓ Pitta ↓ Vata	Heavy, cold, dry	Unripe banana, pomegranate peel, turmeric, blueberries, beans, alfalfa sprouts, lotus seeds

THE EFFECTS OF THE SHADRASAS

Sweet

- Effect on the body: Anabolic, nourishes all the tissues, improves body strength
- Effect on the mind: Compassion, satisfaction
- Effect of overindulgence on the body: Obesity, metabolic problems, heaviness, laziness
- Effect of overindulgence on the mind: Foggy mind
- Effect on the doshas:
    - Has a grounding effect on Vata because of the moisture of the earth and water elements.
    - These same elements give a cooling and soothing effect to Pitta.
    - However, Kapha could become overloaded/aggravated because it already has cool and moist earth and water elements in abundance.

Sour

- Effect on the body: Stimulates salivation, appetite and secretion of digestive juices
- Effect on the mind: Discrimination, comprehension
- Effect of overindulgence on the body: Inflammation, skin disorders, itching, diarrhoea
- Effect of overindulgence on the mind: Hatred and jealousy
- Effect on the doshas:
    - The warmth and humidity of the sour taste exerts a grounding effect on Vata.
    - The excess heat aggravates Pitta.
    - The gentle, moistening aspect can be oppressive to Kapha as it may increase fluid retention and weight.

Salty

- Effect on the body: Improves the flavour of all foods, maintains electrolyte balance in the body
- Effect on the mind: Confidence, zest of life
- Effect of overindulgence on the body: Hair loss, premature greying of hair and wrinkles, oedema, high blood pressure
- Effect of overindulgence on the mind: Hyperactivity
- Effect on the doshas:
    - The warmth of the salty taste helps Vata to hold moisture.
    - The heat of this taste could be counterproductive to Pitta.
    - The warmth liquefies Kapha and hence can promote weight and moisture, therefore aggravating Kapha.

Bitter

- Effect on the body: Suppressor of all other tastes, stimulates digestion, cleanses the liver, scrapes fat and toxins
- Effect on the mind: Detachment from temptation
- Effect of overindulgence on the body: Dryness, emaciation, depletion of body tissues, reduction of libido
- Effect of overindulgence on the mind: Loneliness, inert state of the mind
- Effect on the doshas:
    - The cold, light and dry effect of bitter taste aggravates Vata.
    - The coolness of this taste helps to reduce the heat of Pitta.
    - The light and dry effect of this taste is quite balancing for Kapha.

Pungent

- Effect on the body: Kindles digestive fire, improves digestion and absorption, cleans the mouth, helps in elimination

- Effect on the mind: Boldness, extroversion, focus
- Effect of overindulgence on the body: Burning sensation in the body, heartburn, ulcer, diarrhoea, skin disorders
- Effect of overindulgence on the mind: Anger, irritability, aggressiveness
- Effect on the doshas:
    - The light and drying effect of pungent taste can aggravate Vata because of the extra movement and dehydrating effect on the body.
    - The heat and lightness of this taste aggravates Pitta.
    - The heat, dryness and lightness of this taste has a balancing effect on Kapha.

Astringent

- Effect on the body: Improves absorption and bowel-binding property, scrapes fat
- Effect on the mind: Introversion, grounding
- Effect of overindulgence on the body: Dryness, constipation
- Effect of overindulgence on the mind: Nervousness, anxiety, insomnia
- Effect on the doshas:
    - It chills and dries Vata because of its cool and dry qualities.
    - Its gentle coolness moderates the heat of Pitta.
    - Its dry quality helps balance Kapha.

5

PRAKRITI: YOUR CONSTITUTION

'There's only one me, the closest person that looks like me is my shadow and it's still not me.'

—Eduvie Donald

The biological system integrates the five elements (space, air, fire, water and earth) into three primary energetic patterns known as Tridosha (three doshas). Vata, Pitta and Kapha are the three doshas present in every cell and are essential components of life.

Each of us possesses all three doshas, but in varying proportions. This unique combination of the three doshas determines the distinctive qualities of your mind and body—your prakriti. Prakriti is like a genetic blueprint that remains constant throughout your life. It cannot be altered and holds foremost importance in Ayurveda from both preventative and treatment aspects.

One size does not fit all—everything is personal. Your body's needs vary based on your prakriti, which is why Ayurveda recommends a personalized diet and lifestyle that aligns with your unique constitution. Following a diet and lifestyle suited to your prakriti can help prevent

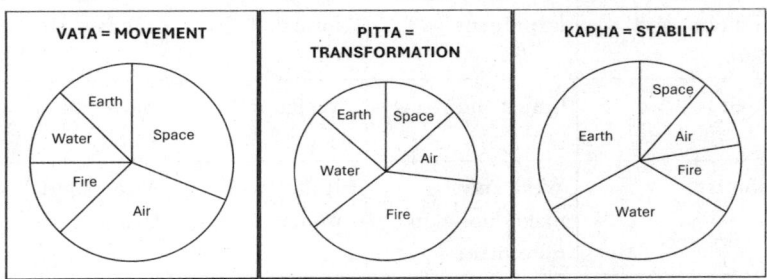

or reduce your susceptibility to prakriti-related diseases. Knowing your constitution is the first step towards comprehending Ayurvedic guidelines and applying them in your daily life for long-term good health.

Self-Assessment of Prakriti

Use this self-assessment chart to understand your prakriti. Circle the answer that is most appropriate to you and your body.

Subject Questions	Answers		
	Vata	*Pitta*	*Kapha*
Body build	Lean	Medium	Well-built
Skin	Dry and rough	Soft and prone to acne	Smooth and moist
Hair	Dry and rough with split ends	Thin and silky	Oily and thick
Complexion	Dull	Radiant	Pale
Eyes	Small	Medium	Big
Eyebrow	Scanty	Thin	Thick
Forehead	Narrow	Medium	Broad
Nails	Small and rough	Thin and soft	Big and smooth
Teeth	Irregular/variable size (big or small)	Medium-sized	Large
Tendons and veins	Prominent	Normal	Well covered
Gait	Quick and fast	Average and steady	Slow and stable
Joints	Weak and makes noise on movement	Healthy with optimal strength	Strong and heavy

EAT ACCORDING TO YOUR BODY TYPE

Subject Questions	Answers		
	Vata	*Pitta*	*Kapha*
Body temperature	Less than normal, with cold hands and feet	Slightly above normal	Normal
Energy	Low	Medium	Excellent
Hunger	Variable and scanty	Strong, sharp	Can skip a meal easily
Habit of eating food	Fast without chewing properly	Eats at moderate speed	Eats slowly and chews food properly
Bowel movements	Dry, hard and scanty; generally once a day or a few times a week	Soft, smooth, yellowish and frequent; generally 2 to 4 times a day	Thick, heavy and large quantity; generally 1 to 2 times a day
Thirst	Variable	Abundant	Less
Perspiration	Not specific	Profuse, sometimes with bad body odour	Less
Sleep	Light sleep and easily interrupted	Sound sleep but short duration	Deep and long sleep
Body weight	Low, difficult to put on weight	Medium, can easily lose or gain weight	Heavy, difficult to lose weight
Memory	Short term is good but not long term	Average	Long term is good
Grasping power	Grasps quickly but not completely and forgets quickly	Grasps quickly and completely and has a good memory	Grasps late and retains for a long time

Subject Questions	Answers		
	Vata	*Pitta*	*Kapha*
Mood	Frequent changes	Changes slowly	Stable/constant
Nature	Jealous and timid	Egoistic and fearless	Grateful and generous
Mental activity	Quick and restless	Smart intellect and aggressive	Calm and stable
Stress tolerance	Poor	Moderate	Good
Reactions under difficult situations	Prone to anxiety and worry	Prone to anger and aggression	Generally calm but sometimes prone to a depressive tendency
Initiative to start any work and pace of performing work	Fast, always in a hurry	Medium, energetic	Slow, steady
Speech	Fast, talkative and inconsistent	Good speakers with argumentative skills	Slow, definite and less speech
Voice	Rough/coarse	Commanding	Deep
Intolerance to weather	Cold	Hot	Good endurance to all weathers
Dreams about	Running, flying, falling, sky and wind	Shining objects, lightning, bright colours, violence, fire and light	Rivers, gardens, swimming, water and greenery

Subject Questions	Answers		
	Vata	*Pitta*	*Kapha*
Physical activity	Very active	Moderate as per need	Less active
Financial habits	Spends money without thinking much	Saves but spends on valuable things	Money-saver, sometimes spends on food
Total	V=	P=	K=
Percentage			
Predominant Dosha			

Count how many you have circled in each dosha (Vata, Pitta and Kapha) category. The highest score of any particular type is the predominant dosha in your prakriti. You may have a mixed result too. That is also okay. It just means that you have a combination type. But you will usually have a dominant dosha.

Now that you have identified which dosha is predominant in your constitution, you can choose the different recipes explained in this book to suit your prakriti. Also, you can adapt the recipes by balancing the flavours and choosing the ingredients that align with your dominant dosha's needs and opting for cooking methods that will be good for you.

FOOD AS MEDICINE

Food is a mahabheshaja, or supreme medicine. Eating the right foods in the right way can help prevent chronic diseases. In fact, food not only supports treatment but, in some cases, can even prevent and treat some diseases. It has the power to complement the treatment of diseases too.

An unsuitable diet is one of the main reasons of imbalance in the doshas. Just as the body is composed of the five elements, food also contains these five elements. Therefore, maintaining balance in your body requires consuming foods that regulate these elements appropriately.

Ayurveda follows a simple yet profound principle: 'Like increases like'. Very simply, this means:

- Foods with properties similar to a dosha will increase that dosha in your body.
- Foods with opposing qualities will help reduce an aggravated dosha.

By adjusting your diet to suit your body's constitution, you can enhance your well-being, support digestion and maintain internal balance. Ayurveda teaches us that aligning our food choices with our prakriti is one of the most effective ways to stay healthy and prevent disease.

Here is a table that illustrates the dosha types and the types of foods that complement them:

Dosha	Natural Properties of Doshas	Properties of Food to Be Used
Vata	Dry Cold Light Rough Mobile	Unctuous Hot Heavy Smooth Stable
Pitta	Hot Sharp Liquid Light	Cold Dull Viscous Heavy
Kapha	Heavy Cold Smooth Dull Unctuous	Light Hot Rough Sharp Dry

EAT ACCORDING TO YOUR BODY TYPE

Dietary Tips for a Vata-Dominant Person

- Prioritize regular eating.
- Eat small portions.
- Take the time to eat slowly; chew the food well.
- Consume warm and nourishing food.
- Food should have more fat and should be seasoned with a variety of spices.
- Consume more cooked food and fewer raw vegetables.
- Avoid too much caffeine and cold foods.
- Include more sweet, sour and salty tastes.
- Drink warm infusions.
- Include more sweet, sour and salty tastes.
- Choose warm over cool, heavy over light and unctuous and moist over dry food.
- Vata plate should be rich in carbs and fat, moderate in proteins and cooked vegetables, minimal or no raw vegetables.

Dietary Tips for a Pitta-Dominant Person

- Eat timely meals and periodic snacks.
- Avoid fasting or long gaps between meals.
- Consume food that is refreshing and cooling in effect.
- Food should have mild flavours or be non-spicy and contain less salt.
- Include moderate fats in your diet.
- Both raw and cooked vegetables are good.
- Very minimal or no use of caffeinated beverages and fermented food.
- Food and drinks should be at room temperature or lukewarm and not hot.
- Include more bitter, sweet and astringent tastes.
- Choose cooling over hot, nourishing over light, mild over acrid or spicy.

- Pitta plate should have equal portions of carbs, vegetables and proteins, cooked with moderate fats and mild or no spices.

Dietary Tips for a Kapha-Dominant Person

- Eat only two to three meals a day.
- Avoid snacking in between meals without actual hunger.
- Practise periodic intermittent fasting.
- Include more raw or grilled vegetables in your diet.
- Use a variety of spices.
- Minimize the intake of sweet and sour tastes, salt, fats, deep-fried food, dairy products, chilled food and drinks.
- Increase the intake of bitter, astringent and pungent tastes.
- Choose light over heavy, warm over cold, dry over oily food.
- Kapha plate should have more vegetables and spices, moderate protein and carbs with minimal fats.

Portion Sizes for Different Prakriti

Prakriti	Portion Size	Ingredients
Vata	Half carbs One-fourth veggies One-fourth proteins	More fats Fewer raw veggies More cooked veggies Moderate spice
Pitta	One-third proteins One-third carbs One-third veggies	Moderate fats Moderate raw veggies Moderate cooked veggies Mild or no spice
Kapha	Half plate of veggies One-fourth carbs One-fourth proteins	Fewer fats Moderate cooked veggies More raw veggies More spice

EAT ACCORDING TO YOUR BODY TYPE

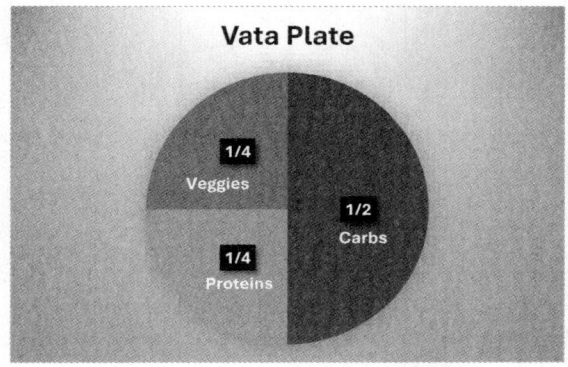

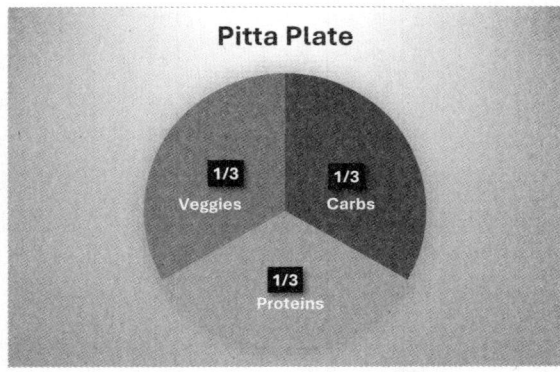

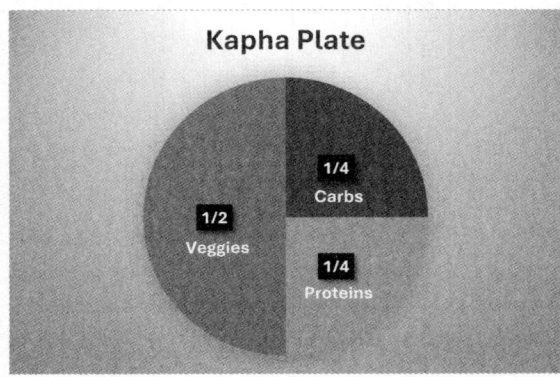

Food Items for Different Prakriti

FOOD	USE / REDUCE	VATA	PITTA	KAPHA
Taste	Use	Sweet, sour and salty tastes	Sweet, bitter and astringent tastes	Pungent, bitter and astringent tastes
	Reduce	Pungent, bitter and astringent tastes	Pungent, sour and salty tastes	Sweet, sour and salty tastes
Qualities	Use	Warm, oily and heavy food	Cool, heavy and dry food	Light, dry and warm food
	Reduce	Light, dry, cold food	Warm, oily and light foods	Heavy, oily and cold food
Grains	Use	Rice, wheat, oats	Rice, wheat, oats, barley	Barley, corn, millets, buckwheat, rye
	Reduce	Barley, millets, buckwheat, rye	Corn, rye, millets	Oats, rice, wheat
Legumes	Use	Mung	Mung, black-eyed peas, chickpeas, split peas, kidney beans	Mung, pink lentils, horse gram, chickpeas, pigeon peas
	Reduce	Chickpeas, black-eyed peas	Pink lentils, yellow lentils	Kidney beans, black lentils

Food Items for Different Prakriti

FOOD	USE / REDUCE	VATA	PITTA	KAPHA
Fruits	Use	Banana, mango, apricot, fig, orange, peach, kiwi, pineapple, coconut	Grapes, melon, cherries, coconut, avocado, mango, pomegranate, fully ripe pineapple, orange, plum	Apple, pear, pomegranate, cranberries, apricot
	Reduce	Dry fruits, apple	Grapefruit, apricot, berries	Banana, avocado, pineapple, orange, coconut, melon, dates, figs
Vegetables	Use	Beets, asparagus, carrot, zucchini	Asparagus, cucumber, potato, sweet potato, green leafy vegetables, pumpkin, broccoli, cauliflower, celery, okra, lettuce, green beans, zucchini	Nightshades
	Reduce	Raw vegetables, cruciferous vegetables, radish, peas	Tomato, hot peppers, carrot, beet, eggplant, onion, garlic, radish, spinach	Sweet potato, tomato, zucchini

Food Items for Different Prakriti

FOOD	USE / REDUCE	VATA	PITTA	KAPHA
Dairy Products	Use	All dairy products	Milk, butter, ghee	Low-fat dairy products
	Reduce	–	Sour, fermented products	Cream, yoghurt
Spices	Use	All spices	Coriander, cardamom, saffron, fennel	All spices
	Reduce	–	Fenugreek, salt, mustard seeds, cayenne	Salt
Oils	Use	All oils, especially sesame oil	Olive, sunflower, coconut oil, ghee	Olive oil, mustard oil, almond oil
	Reduce	Corn oil	Mustard oil, sesame oil	Apricot, walnut, coconut
Nuts and Seeds	Use	Sesame seeds, sunflower seeds, soaked nuts	Almond, chia seeds, pumpkin seeds, sunflower seeds	–
	Reduce	–	Sesame seeds, pecans, pine nuts, cashews	Cashews, pine nuts, peanuts, sesame seeds

Food Items for Different Prakriti

FOOD	USE / REDUCE	VATA	PITTA	KAPHA
Non-Veg	Use	Eggs, goat, bison, buffalo, pork, rabbit, goose, quail, pheasant, dark meat (meat from legs and thighs of chicken and turkey), duck, crab, shellfish (clams, oysters, octopus, mussels, lobster, shrimp), fish such as shark, herring, cod, flatfish, red snapper, tuna, mackerel, sardine and salmon	Egg whites, pheasant, white meat (chicken and turkey breast), lamb, goat, bison, rabbit, quail, mackerel, flatfish, shellfish	White meat, quail, goat, cod, trout, perch, pomfret, shrimp
	Reduce	Quail, white meat, lamb	Egg yolks, dark meat, duck, lamb, pork, goose, buffalo, sardine, tuna, salmon, cod, shark, red snapper, crab	Egg yolks, pheasant, duck, lamb, pork, buffalo, rabbit, goose, sardine, mackerel, red snapper, tuna, salmon, sharks, carp, catfish, pike, shellfish

Food Items for Different Prakriti

FOOD	USE / REDUCE	VATA	PITTA	KAPHA
Sweeteners	Use	Misri (rock sugar), desi khand (muscovado or unrefined sugar with a coarser texture and a darker colour), jaggery (unrefined, concentrated form of sugarcane juice), palm sugar (from the sap of the palmyra palm, date palm, coconut palm or sugar palm), honey, liquid jaggery (molasses)	Misri, desi khand, palm sugar	Honey, liquid jaggery, jaggery
	Reduce	Stevia	Honey, liquid jaggery, jaggery	Misri, desi khand, palm sugar

6

EAT FOR YOUR MIND

'If you can change your mind, you can change your life.'
—William James

The mind is a micro entity that plays a major role in maintaining good health by guiding the right dietary habits, sleep discipline and exercise routine. The mind differentiates between right and wrong through thought processes based on input from your sense organs. Most diseases are caused by the injudicious use of your sense organs and a lack of control over the mind. While the sense organs are made to receive their respective subjects, it is the mind that indulges in them. Hence, if you can control the activity of your mind, you can avoid disease, pain and grief, and live a peaceful and healthy life.

Just like the doshas of your body, the mind also has gunas (properties). The five elements combine to create three gunas of the mind. Unlike the prakriti of your body, which cannot be altered, the gunas of your mind can be altered through diet and lifestyle practices. Thus, the three gunas have a direct impact on your mind, while the three doshas influence your mind indirectly.

Your mind and intellect depend on the three gunas, and they play an important role in decision-making regarding all aspects of life, including the consumption of wholesome or unwholesome diets, behaviour, emotions and lifestyle. So a healthy mind and intellect will help you remain physically and psychologically happy and fit. The mind and intellect should always be given due importance in both the preventive and curative aspects of physical and psychological disorders. Unlike prakriti, the mind and intellect can be modified, educated and improved. Everything you eat, think and do exerts a positive or negative impact on the mind and intellect, thus influencing your health. The balanced state of the three gunas is the key to a long and healthy life, and Ayurveda leads you to this key.

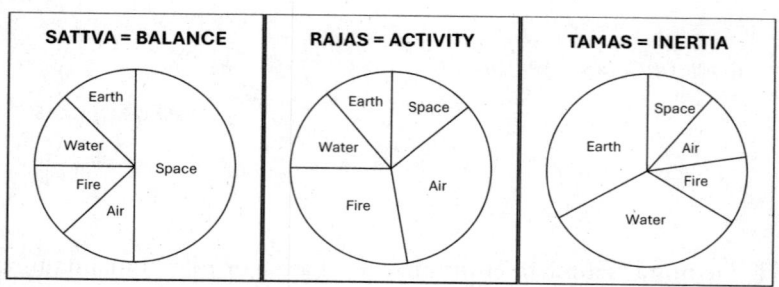

The three gunas are Sattva, Rajas and Tamas. Sattva, Rajas and Tamas are the tendencies of mind, body and consciousness. They describe our behaviour, thoughts and health. Below are the characteristics of these three gunas.

- Sattva is a state of balance, harmony and stability. It gives rise to health and happiness. It makes you enthusiastic and non-egoistic. Success or failure will have no effect on you, as it makes the mind more conscious.
- Feelings of longing and attachment are characteristic of the Rajas guna. Rajas is concerned with dynamic activity. It prompts hasty decisions, makes you passionate for power and causes disequilibrium. Rajas alters the perception of your mind, making false impressions of the external world seem real. This may temporarily cause happiness but in the long run, you will lose inner peace. Desires and emotional upsets are caused by Rajas.
- Tamas leads to inertia. It dulls the mind. The actions of a Tamasic person are more unsteady as it causes agitation and delusions in the mind. Ignorance arises from Tamas.

An adequate balance of the three gunas is essential, as Sattva balances the energy of Rajas while providing stability through Tamas. If your manas (mind) is dominated by Sattva, you will have a more positive attitude. A balanced Rajas makes you more active and competitive, while a small proportion of Tamas provides stability. Higher proportions of Rajas and Tamas are responsible for a more negative attitude. This is why Ayurveda emphasizes a vegetarian diet cooked with love and eaten mindfully—to increase Sattva in the mind. Adopting a Sattvic diet and a healthy lifestyle from an early age is a step towards personalized preventative care, offering anti-ageing and rejuvenating benefits. It boosts your immunity, thereby leading to a healthy, disease-free, more productive and high-quality life.

A Sattva diet has a positive effect on health, whereas a diet that increases Rajas and Tamas destroys the body–mind equilibrium and feeds the body at the expense of the mind. A Rajas-dominant diet increases anger, irritation, anxiety, stress and restlessness, and living on a Tamas-dominant diet leads to metabolic problems, depression, laziness, attachment, etc.

A Sattvic diet is a fresh vegetarian diet that is free from additives and preservatives, light to digest and agreeable to the body. It not only nourishes the body but promotes mental clarity as well. A Rajasic diet gives a burst of energy, but overindulgence in it eventually increases stress and leads to anger and irritation. A Tamasic diet has a grounding effect on the body and mind but too much intake of a Tamasic diet makes a person lazy and inactive.

The characteristics of the different prakritis and the corresponding gunas are summarized below.

VATA		
SATTVA QUALITIES	RAJAS QUALITIES	TAMAS QUALITIES
• Positive mental energy	• Hyperactive	• Fearful
• Adaptive	• Agitated	• Dishonest
• Quick comprehension	• Indecisive	• Self-destructive

PITTA		
SATTVA QUALITIES	RAJAS QUALITIES	TAMAS QUALITIES
• Perceptive • Courageous • Friendly • Leadership qualities	• Egoistic • Impulsive • Manipulative • Aggressive	• Violent • Vengeful

KAPHA		
SATTVA QUALITIES	RAJAS QUALITIES	TAMAS QUALITIES
• Calm • Supportive • Nurturing • Loyal	• Materialistic • Attachment • Greed • Sentimental	• Lethargic • Dull • Insensitive • Apathetic

That Which Increases Sattva	That Which Increases Rajas	That Which Increases Tamas
• Eating consciously and in moderation • Wholesome, nutritious and calming food with a balance of all tastes • Herbal infusions • Ghee, organic milk • Fresh fruits and vegetables that are seasonal • Vegetarian diet	• Hurried eating • Excess intake of garlic, chillies, onion, mustard, spicy, salty and hot food • Excess consumption of coffee, tea, caffeinated beverages • Excess intake of chicken and fish	• Overeating and frequent eating • Excess intake of chilled food, stale food, heavy-to- digest food, refrigerated and reheated food • Excess consumption of cold drinks, ice creams and chocolates • Overconsumption of alcohol • Red meat intake in excess

A Sattvic diet makes you feel more connected to the universe. It is the need of the hour, given the rise in stress and lifestyle diseases. This diet promotes wellness and plays a crucial role in preserving health and preventing diseases because it is nutrient-dense, thus improving digestion and cellular nutrition, nourishing the body and calming the mind.

7

EAT ACCORDING TO THE SEASON AND THE TIME OF THE DAY

'The joy of eating seasonally is the joy of fresh produce and fresh foods.'

—Anna Lappé

According to Ayurveda, the strength of your digestive fire is influenced by the position of the sun. The higher the position of the sun, the stronger your digestive fire. Therefore, it is best to eat heavy foods at midday, while your dinner should be light and breakfast should be moderate.

Imagine drinking a hot and spicy soup for lunch in summer. Would you enjoy it when you're already hot and sweaty? Likely not—because your body's doshic state varies with each season. As such, your diet must be adapted to the season, considering its effect on your body, prakriti, and the state of your digestive fire. In other words, you need to choose foods that support your agni and balance the doshas prone to aggravation in a particular season—without disturbing the inherent equilibrium of the doshas in your prakriti. This explains why a standard diet is not suitable for maintaining good health throughout the year. As the seasons change, your body's needs change too.

Different seasons exert different effects on the body. If your body is unable to adapt to seasonal stressors, it could lead to a doshic imbalance, making you susceptible to various diseases. You must live in harmony with nature, otherwise your immunity may be compromised, increasing your risk of contracting lifestyle diseases.

> It is beneficial to practise intermittent fasting in spring. In winter, one should consume satisfying and nourishing foods; in summer, opt for cooling and sweet foods; and during the monsoon, eat warm and light meals.

SPRING

Status of Doshas
Kapha ++
Pitta -
Vata -

Status of Agni – Moderate

Selection of Food – Hot potency food that is light to digest and less unctuous in nature

Recommended Tastes – Bitter, pungent and astringent

Indicated – Old grains, especially barley and wheat, honey, spinach, lettuce, mustard greens, peas, turnips, broccoli, artichokes, spring onions, coriander, cumin, garlic, turmeric and fennel

Contraindicated – Cold, heavy, viscous foods, and sour and sweet tastes

SUMMER

Status of Doshas
Vata +
Pitta -
Kapha -

Status of Agni – Weak

Selection of Food – Light to digest and unctuous food, and drinks that are cooling in nature

Recommended Tastes – Sweet

Indicated – Juicy fruits and vegetables, coconut water, fennel/mint infusion, sugarcane juice, milk, sweet yoghurt, raisins, sherbet berry, cucumber, celery, leafy greens and asparagus

Contraindicated – Hot and spicy food, sour tastes, excess salt, mustard, fresh ginger and garlic

EAT ACCORDING TO YOUR BODY TYPE

MONSOON

Status of Doshas: Vata ++, Pitta +, Kapha -	Status of Agni – Weak	Selection of Food – Hot and unctuous food
Recommended Tastes – Sweet, sour and salty	Indicated – Thin soups, whey, asafoetida, pepper, ginger and old grains	Contraindicated – Raw or undercooked, heavy-to-digest and cold food

AUTUMN

Status of Doshas: Pitta ++, Vata -, Kapha -	Status of Agni – Moderate	Selection of Food – Less unctuous and easy-to-digest food
Recommended Tastes – Sweet, astringent and bitter	Indicated – Rice, green leafy vegetables, berries, plums, ghee, milk, cane sugar, honey and mung beans	Contraindicated – Sour and alkaline tastes, hot and heavy-to-digest food, yoghurt

WINTER

Status of Doshas: Kapha +, Pitta -, Vata -	Status of Agni – Good	Selection of Food – Hot potency food that is unctuous and heavy to digest
Recommended Tastes – Sweet, sour and salty	Indicated – Fermented food like sauerkraut, kimchi, etc., pumpkin, spinach, potatoes, carrots, beets, onions, apples, oranges, kiwis, grapes, dates, dairy products, black lentils, rice, wheat and freshly harvested corn	Contraindicated – Cold, light and dry food

EATING ACCORDING TO THE TIME OF THE DAY

The rules for eating food at different times of the day are explained in Ayurveda based on the diurnal variations that influence the dosha status during different periods. According to Ayurvedic principles, one should have a moderate breakfast before 8 a.m. (as Kapha dominates in the morning hours), a big lunch at midday or before 1 p.m. (as Pitta is strong during this time) and a light and early dinner, preferably before sunset or at least by 7.30 p.m. (as Kapha becomes strong after sunset).

A balanced breakfast: Break the fast (as we do not eat for about twelve hours at night) by eating a moderate meal. As your digestive fire is relatively low because of the long night of rest, your body may struggle to digest a heavy breakfast. Warm porridge is a nutritious breakfast option in Ayurvedic practice. You can enjoy different porridges (rice, mung, barley, millet) with various nuts, dried fruits, seeds, and milk or yoghurt. Alternatively, you can opt for a variety of warm, nutritious and light breakfast foods. Coffee, tea and white bread are definitely not nutritious so you should avoid these. An ideal breakfast typically consists of fibres, protein and healthy fats.

Breakfast is not mandatory for a Kapha-dominant person or someone suffering from metabolic problems. In such cases, brunch is a better option. But remember, skip breakfast only if doing so leaves you feeling physically better and mentally alert.

Mid-morning snack: If you are a Vata or Pitta person, you may enjoy a cup of yoghurt or a fruit two or two-and-a-half hours after breakfast.

Large lunch: Enjoy your largest meal at lunchtime, when your digestive strength is at its peak and the external heat (sunlight) supports digestion. It is ideal to include all the macronutrients—carbohydrates, proteins, vegetables and healthy fats. If you consume meat, lunch is the best time to do so.

Mid-evening snack: Roasted nuts or a fruit can be a healthy snack around three hours after lunch along with a cup of a warm herbal infusion. However, if you are Kapha-dominant, it's better to skip the evening snack.

Downsized dinner: Dinner should be light and easy to digest, as physical activity reduces in the evening and there is no external heat to aid digestion. Since Kapha becomes dominant after sunset, aim to eat dinner before sunset or by 7.30 p.m. at the latest. You may skip simple carbohydrates at dinner as your energy demands reduce. Instead, focus on vegetarian proteins, vegetables, fats, and a small portion of whole grains. Avoid yoghurt, cheese, eggs, meat, or heavy-to-digest foods such as pastries and ice cream at night, as they are heavy and impair digestion.

In today's world, many people have a rushed breakfast, a packed lunch, and their biggest meal is dinner. This reversal contributes to lifestyle diseases. The common excuse is lack of time in the morning—grabbing a quick bite or leftovers for lunch or eating from the office canteen. In contrast, dinner becomes a well-prepared, comforting and heavy meal. This happens for several reasons—you have more time in the evening, meals become family bonding experiences, and social events often take place over dinner. All of this stems from poor time management. With proper weekly planning, grocery organization, and menu preparation, you can enjoy healthy, balanced meals with your family.

8

TEN RULES TO EAT HEALTHIER

'Your body is the direct result of what you eat as well as what you don't eat.'

—Gloria Swanson

A majority of the foundational texts of Ayurveda such as the *Charaka Samhita* and *Susrutha Samhita* have outlined rules for food intake under the section 'Ahara Vidhi Viseshaayatana', which details the principles for selection, preparation and consumption of food. Here are ten rules that everyone can follow:

1. Food that is warm or hot is delicious and ideal for consumption. Eating warm food stimulates our digestive fire, thus facilitating the proper and timely digestion of food.
2. Unctuous food increases the plumpness of the body, nourishes the tissues and promotes strength. Hence unctuous food should be part of one's diet. Even if you are eating a vegetable salad, add some olive oil or sprinkle seeds on it to add extra nourishment.
3. Food should be taken in proper quantities to help promote longevity and balance all three doshas.
4. Eat food only when the previous meal is digested. If you eat food before the previous meal is digested, the digestive products from the previous meal get mixed with the food taken afterwards, resulting in an imbalance of all three doshas.

5. You should avoid the intake of food with contradictory properties because it may give rise to diseases.

6. Eating in a pleasant environment with comfortable seating makes the eating experience an enjoyable one as it minimizes distractions, deepens the appreciation for the meal and helps you fully engage all your senses in the experience, thus promoting a holistic approach to nourishment that extends beyond physical health, positively impacting your mental and emotional well-being as well.

7. Food should not be eaten hurriedly. When you eat quickly or hurriedly, you may not masticate (chew) the food properly and this affects your digestion. You fail to relish the taste of food when you are in a hurry.

8. Eating food too slowly will not give you proper satisfaction, hence you might end up eating more or less than what is actually required by your body. Additionally, the food becomes cold due to slow consumption, which is not ideal.

9. You should eat mindfully without talking or laughing or dealing with any distractions. Research shows that proper mastication can facilitate salivary secretion.[7] Eating while being distracted by television, excessive conversation or reading can prevent you from maximizing your nutrition. When you are distracted, you do not chew your food properly and when partially masticated food enters the stomach, it is forced to digest this. So, you should always eat mindfully.

10. You should eat food in a prescribed manner with due regard to yourself, that is, to eat food that is good for your prakriti and according to the season and the time of the day.

9

FOUNDATIONAL AYURVEDIC FOODS AND HOW TO PREPARE THEM

'Simple ingredients prepared in a simple way – that's the best way to take your everyday cooking to a higher level.'
—Jose Andres

All the necessary nutrients for our body are supplied by different food classes. Food articles known as 'ahara dravyas' are mainly categorized into two groups—food (ahara dravyas) and drinks (drava dravyas). The first category deals with solid/hard food articles that require mastication, like cereals, vegetables, pulses, etc., whereas the second one deals with all liquids like water, milk, soups, juices, etc. The two categories combined are called 'Annapana' (anna meaning 'food' and pana meaning 'drinks'). All the classical textbooks of Ayurveda explain food classification (ahara varga). The *Charaka Samhita* talks about food and drinks in one chapter, whereas the *Susrutha Samhita* and *Ashtanga Sangraha* detail food and drinks separately as two chapters.

The *Charaka Samhita* lists twelve food groups with different nutritional values, which are explained in the table below:

Annapana Varga	Food Group in English	Nutritional Value	Examples
Shookadhanya	Cereals	Rich source of carbohydrates	Rice, millets, barley, wheat

Annapana Varga	Food Group in English	Nutritional Value	Examples
Shamidhanya	Pulses and legumes	Rich in protein	Mung, black gram, chickpeas, pigeon peas
Mamsa varga	Flesh and meat	Good source of proteins, minerals and fats	Crab, fish, chicken
Shaaka varga	Vegetables	Rich in roughage, antioxidants, vitamins and minerals	Spinach, chillies, ash gourd
Phala varga	Fruits	Rich in carbohydrates, antioxidants, vitamins, minerals and electrolytes	Pomegranate, grapes, dates, mango, citron
Harita varga	Class of greens, salads	Rich in roughage, vitamins and minerals	Fresh ginger, radish, lemon, basil, coriander, onion, garlic
Madhya varga	Alcoholic beverages	Rich in antioxidants and carbohydrates	Fermented drinks prepared from sugarcane juice, grapes, finger millet
Jala varga	Water	Hydrates the body, is rich in minerals and is an elixir	Rainwater and water from ponds, wells, lakes, rivers

Annapana Varga	Food Group in English	Nutritional Value	Examples
Gorasa varga	Milk and milk products	Rich in fats, proteins, carbohydrates	Milk, yoghurt, butter, buttermilk, ghee
Ikshu varga	Sugarcane products	Carbohydrate source	Jaggery, molasses, desi khand
Krutanna varga	Class of recipes, food preparations	Good source of functional components such as proteins, vitamins, minerals and phytochemicals	Manda (gruel water), peya (gruel), juices, soups
Ahara upayogi	Class of accessory food articles/ food adjuvants	Improves taste and aroma, rich source of antioxidants	Oil, dry ginger, black pepper, asafoetida, rock salt

Every food category comprises a range of items that share similar nutritional characteristics, and each category contributes significantly to a balanced diet. Certain food categories are additionally divided into subcategories to highlight foods that are especially rich in specific vitamins and minerals.

However, as per origin, food can be classified as plant-based or animal-based.

SPICES

> *'Use spices for flavour in food rather than adding a bunch of oils, fats, or sauces.'*
> —Marisol Nichols

Spices have been used in cooking and medicine from time immemorial. They improve the flavour, aroma, colour and taste of food. When used with knowledge, spices can help balance your meals. By modifying spice combinations, the same dish can be adapted to suit different prakritis. Since most spices support digestion, they help reduce or prevent ama in the body. If you want to protect yourself from acute and chronic diseases, include spices in your daily diet. The good news? Spices are low in calories and free from added sugars and sodium. Here are some of the health benefits of spices:

- They are a rich source of antioxidants.
- They are appetizing and carminative.
- They boost digestion and help balance food cravings.
- They improve metabolism and energize the body.
- They have anti-inflammatory and antimicrobial properties.
- They improve brain function, enhance immunity and keep the body healthy.
- They help treat/prevent colic pain.

How to Use Spices in Your Diet[9]

- **Infusions:** Who does not love to sip a hot infusion on a rainy day? Ginger or basil-ginger infusions are common home remedies for a cold or cough. Infusions also offer many health benefits and can replace tea or coffee. Each spice has a unique effect: ginger is stimulating, cardamom is calming, cumin aids digestion, and basil helps liquefy phlegm. Spices like fennel and coriander contain volatile oils that evaporate if heated above 25°C, so they're best used in cold infusions. Fennel helps with acidity, and coriander with water retention.

How to make a hot infusion

Crush ¼ teaspoon of a whole spice using a mortar and pestle or grinder. Add it to a tea infuser and steep in hot water for 5–7 minutes. If you don't have a tea infuser, steep the spice directly in hot water, cover, then strain.

How to make a cold infusion

Make a coarse powder of whole spices as in the hot infusion preparation method. Now take a cup of water (at room temperature), add ¼ tsp of the crushed spice, cover with a lid and leave it overnight or for 5 to 6 hours. Then filter and drink the infusion. If the weather is cold and if you prefer to have something warm, you can heat the water a bit just before filtering it. Enjoy the infusion.

- **Flavoured drinks:** Lavender and mint are used for flavouring summer drinks. Ginger can be added to lemon water.
- **Vegetable/fruit salad dressing:** Spices such as ginger, parsley, dill, garlic, marjoram, thyme and chives are used as vegetable salad dressing and spices such as black pepper, cumin, star anise and cinnamon are used as fruit salad dressing. Spices help improve the digestion of salads.
- **Direct consumption:** Chewing of fennel seeds after a meal helps neutralize acids. Chewing cardamom seeds helps to get rid of bad breath.
- **Food additives:** Spices such as cinnamon, cardamom and nutmeg are used to infuse ghee, oil, jam, candies, etc., to add flavour.
- **Fortification of dairy products:** Milk can be spiced with cardamom, cinnamon, saffron, nutmeg and turmeric. Buttermilk can be spiced with cumin, asafoetida, ginger, thyme, mint and mustard. Yoghurt can be spiced with cardamom, cinnamon, coriander, chives or turmeric. In addition to adding flavour, the spices enhance the nutritional value of dairy products.

- **Food adjuncts:** Spices make food tastier and flavourful. They increase hunger and have therapeutic benefits too. Fenugreek and turmeric help regulate blood sugar levels. Garlic, black pepper and onion help to lower cholesterol levels. Dry ginger helps with arthritis because of its anti-inflammatory properties. Cinnamon helps to reduce body weight. Turmeric, ginger, garlic and black pepper possess antioxidant properties and have cancer-prevention potential. Garlic has a cardioprotective effect. Cardamom and nutmeg help to relieve stress.[10]
- **As adjuvants:** Many spices are used for seasoning food. Spices such as asafoetida, cumin, mustard, garlic and ginger are used for tempering lentils. Rosemary, bay leaf, sage, thyme, basil, cinnamon, marjoram, mace and onion are used for seasoning soups.
- **Garnishing desserts:** Spices like mace, anise, cloves, cinnamon and cardamom are used for garnishing desserts as they enhance the taste as well as aid in better digestion.
- **Preservatives:** Some spices are used to increase the shelf life of food products. Turmeric and black pepper are used to prevent raw meat from getting spoiled by microbial growth. Salt, cumin and mustard seeds are added to pickles to preserve them.

OILS IN COOKING

Just like carbohydrates and proteins, fats are also important for your body. According to Ayurveda, healthy fats are homologous to ojas or cellular immunity. Fats provide nourishment to your body cells. In simple words, fat is used as fuel by the body. If fat is not converted into energy it is simply stored by the body in fat cells for usage at a later time when food might be scarce and your body needs energy. The cell membrane is made up of a selectively permeable lipid bilayer, a protective barrier that also maintains the integrity of the cell. Healthy fats are lipophilic, so they easily dissolve in the lipid bilayer and enter the cells. Our brain is also composed of 60 per cent fat; hence, for the preservation of brain integrity and mental and cognitive functions, you should include a sufficient amount of healthy fats in your diet.[11]

To know the different healthy and unhealthy fats available in food, you should understand the different types of fats first.

- Saturated fat is healthy because it is natural and stable upon heating. Hence it can be used for cooking. Some examples are butter, ghee and coconut oil.
- Unsaturated fats are also natural but undergo some processing, hence they are unstable for cooking. However, they can be used as a dressing or added to food at low temperatures. Some examples are avocado oil, olive oil, walnut and flaxseed oil.
- Hydrogenated/trans fats are highly unnatural as they undergo extensive processing. They are not good for consumption. Some examples are vegetable shortening, margarine and vanaspati.

Ayurveda suggests the use of filtered oils for cooking. As the nutrient value of refined oil is low, you should avoid it.

- Ghee, mustard oil, sesame oil and coconut oil are good for deep frying as they have a high smoke point.
- Oils of peanut and sunflower can be used for cooking.
- Olive oil, flaxseed oil, almond oil and hemp seed oil should be used only as dressings.

To use the right cooking oil for you and your family, you have to evaluate your prakriti/body constitution first.

- If you are a Vata person, you will be very active physically but prone to dry intestines, skin and hair. As you tend to have cold extremities and susceptibility to aches and pains, cooking oils that are highly unctuous and heating in nature will be beneficial for you.
- Pitta persons are very fast and active. If you are a Pitta person, you will have increased body heat and will be vulnerable to skin problems

and hyperacidity, so cooking oils that have a sweet taste and cooling properties are suitable for you.
- If you are a Kapha person, you will have a slow metabolism and a tendency to develop metabolic problems as you are normally not a very physically active person. So, cooking oils that are heating and light in nature should be used by you.

OILS AND THE DOSHAS	
Oils	**Action on Doshas**
Ghee	Reduces Vata and Pitta Does not increase Kapha
Sesame oil	Reduces Vata and Kapha Slightly increases Pitta
Coconut oil	Reduces Vata and Pitta Increases Kapha
Mustard oil	Reduces Kapha and Vata Increases Pitta
Groundnut oil	Reduces Vata Increases Pitta
Olive oil	Reduces Kapha and Vata
Sunflower oil	Reduces Vata and Pitta Okay for Kapha
Almond oil	Reduces Vata Increases Pitta
Flaxseed oil	Reduces Vata Increases Pitta and Kapha
Hemp seed oil	Reduces Vata and Pitta

- Hydrogenated oil is harmful to the body. Cooking with sesame oil, coconut oil or ghee is the best. According to Ayurveda, sesame oil is nutritious, whereas safflower oil is unwholesome. Ayurveda also suggests avoiding reheating oils. A lot of oil is used for deep frying, and many of us do not want to waste it, so we reuse the oil for cooking. But most oils, especially corn, soybean and sunflower oil, when reheated can form 4-hydroxy-trans-2-nonenal (HNE), which is associated with the risk of cardiovascular diseases, liver diseases, cancer, etc.[12] Hence reheating oils that have been used for deep frying is not a good practice.

- Cold-pressed oils have become popular in recent years. The slow cold-pressed method does not use heat or chemicals; hence it preserves the nutrients and antioxidants in the oil. The traditional wooden extraction machine has now been replaced by hydraulic oil press machines, which also alter the nutrient content of the oil.

GHEE

Ghee is found in every Indian household. It is used widely for cooking, dressing, massaging the skin and hair and in lighting lamps for prayers. Ghee is believed to bring positivity and prosperity, which is why ghee lamps are popular in India. The aromatic flavour and richness of ghee make it the best choice for desserts and creamy gravies.

Ghee is an important dietary ingredient suitable for people of all ages. Ghee has high nutritional value and is widely recommended in Ayurvedic texts. Unlike the other cooking oils, the potency of ghee increases with its age—the older the ghee, the higher its therapeutic benefits. There are many ways to use ghee—oral intake, nasal application, as eye drops, external use for massage, rectal administration in the form of an enema, etc.

How to Prepare Ghee

- Take a cup of milk cream. You can use store-bought cream or collect cream at home from boiled milk. Store-bought cream will definitely not have the same nutritional value as that of cream collected at home. Every day, when you boil milk and allow it to cool down to room temperature, it will form a creamy layer on top. Collect this cream in a container and store it in the refrigerator. Keep doing this every day until you get 1 cup of cream. Less than 1 cup of cream will not be enough to make ghee.

- Add 1 tsp of yoghurt (preferably sour) to 1 cup of milk cream and leave it at room temperature for 24 to 48 hours (depending on the weather) so it gets fermented. In the summer, you have to leave this at room temperature for 24 hours; in the winter you can leave this in a hot area (say on your terrace under the sun or in your kitchen near the gas stove) for 48 hours. The cream will develop a tangy smell because of the fermentation.
- Now add ½ cup of slightly cold water and churn well using a wooden whisk or electric hand blender to separate the butter from the residual liquid (buttermilk). If you use a wooden whisk, you may have to churn the mixture for 5 to 7 minutes and if you use an electric hand blender you may have to whisk it for only 1 to 2 minutes. Be careful not to whisk the butter too much when you use an electric hand blender.
- Now use a fine mesh sieve to strain the butter. You can line the sieve with a cheesecloth if you wish. Then rinse the butter using cold water. This helps to rinse off residual buttermilk so as to remove the sour taste (created due to fermentation) and to improve the shelf life of the butter. Let all the water drain from the butter.
- Transfer the butter to a thick-bottomed kadai and heat it on a moderate flame. Once the butter melts, the milk solids will begin to cook and a white foam will slowly rise to the surface. Now start stirring the melted butter gently to prevent the milk solids from sticking to the bottom of the vessel. When the milk solids start to turn light brown and emit a nutty flavour, switch off the gas stove. As the vessel will be hot, the milk solids will continue to cook and become deep brown. Make sure not to burn the milk solids as it will decrease the nutrients. Then filter the ghee. Place a cheesecloth or filter paper on a steel mesh strainer and put this strainer on a dry glass vessel or stainless steel container. Now pour the ghee into the cheesecloth or filter paper to remove the brownish milk solids and collect the ghee

in the vessel. Let it cool down to room temperature and then cover the vessel with a lid. Ghee prepared in this Ayurvedic way will not increase serum cholesterol levels.

How to Store Ghee

Once prepared, store the ghee in a moisture-free airtight container, preferably a glass container. You can store ghee at room temperature in all seasons; there is no need to refrigerate it. But keep it away from direct sunlight. It is normal for ghee to liquify in hot weather and solidify in cold weather. If you prepare ghee properly in the above-mentioned way, it will only have negligible amounts of lactose and is therefore acceptable/safe to consume by people who have lactose intolerance or a milk allergy.

The Benefits of Ghee

Ghee is a sweet substance that is congenial to all body types. Ghee is considered to be 'yogavahi', meaning it has a unique capacity to assimilate the properties of other substances into it and is, therefore, of great medicinal value. It imparts the benefits of essential fatty acids, improves digestion, nourishes the body's tissues, improves the voice, strengthens the sense organs, enhances immunity, increases longevity, helps to regulate body weight, removes fatigue, improves intellect and memory, relieves dryness in the body (in the skin, hair and intestines as well), heals ulcers and wounds, improves vision, is good for the skin, has a moistening and cooling effect on the body, strengthens bones, and helps in pregnancy as it is nourishing and enlivening.

Ghee is ideal for people of Vata and Pitta body types as it calms down both Vata and Pitta. It is okay for the Kapha body type.

Consuming Ghee

Always consume ghee with warm liquids, preferably before meals or with meals. You can take a teaspoon of ghee with warm water before meals. You may add ghee to warm soups/milk/herbal infusions or mix it with rice/vegetables, or apply it on toast. If you are a person with strong digestion and a good appetite then you can eat ghee in good quantities, whereas if you tend to have weak digestion or a low appetite, you should consume ghee in small quantities. You should not consume ghee immediately after eating food or during indigestion or fever. Also, you should not have it with cold substances such as cold water or cold milk.

Ghee is a nectar when used in an optimal quantity according to one's digestive capacity and health needs.

YOGHURT

Yoghurt is made by fermenting milk with a yoghurt culture. To make yoghurt at home, follow these steps:

- Boil 4 cups of milk in a saucepan.
- When it is lukewarm (slightly above body temperature), transfer 4 cups of milk to a stainless-steel vessel and add 2 tsp yoghurt (from previous yoghurt/commercial yoghurt). Stir gently and cover with a lid.
- Leave it undisturbed for 8 to 10 hours.
- In cold climates, wrap a woollen cloth around the vessel and keep it in a warm place. Or you can use a hotpot instead of a stainless-steel vessel to make yoghurt. In summer or warm weather, a wrap or hotpot is not needed.

Once prepared, yoghurt is good for consumption when it is fresh, or you can refrigerate it and consume it within 24 to 48 hours. To maintain a healthy digestive system, make sure to keep the yoghurt out of the refrigerator and let it come to room temperature before consumption. Yoghurt is best consumed in the daytime. Avoid consuming it at night. If yoghurt becomes sour it is not good for direct consumption; however, it can be used to cook certain dishes that will help support healthy digestion by modulating the gut microbiota. Ayurveda says to avoid daily consumption of yoghurt in the seasons of summer, autumn and spring, and if you suffer from Kapha disorders such as sinusitis, respiratory allergy, increased sleep, weight gain, etc., or increased Pitta issues such as inflammatory skin conditions (acne, eczema and urticaria).

It is ideal to consume yoghurt with any of the following to prevent an imbalance of the doshas: rock salt, cane sugar, honey, black pepper, ghee, or mung.

The Benefits of Yoghurt

- 1 cup of yoghurt + 1 tbsp of cane sugar powder → Balances Vata and Pitta doshas
- 1 cup of yoghurt + 1 tbsp of jaggery powder → Balances Vata dosha
- 1 cup of yoghurt + powders of black pepper, dry ginger and mustard (¼ tsp each) → Balances Kapha and improves digestion as well

BUTTERMILK

Buttermilk is nothing but churned and diluted yoghurt. Ayurveda recommends its daily consumption in winter and for conditions such as indigestion, irritable bowel syndrome, colicky pain and low appetite. Its consumption should be reduced in hot weather and during the postpartum period.

In fermented products like yoghurt and buttermilk, most of the lactose is converted to lactic acid or acetic acid by the enzymes of the fermenting bacteria, hence these are not only easy to digest but have health benefits too. They replenish the friendly bacteria in the gut flora. We can make buttermilk easily at home using yoghurt.

Based on the fat content, buttermilk can be classified into three types:

1. **No-fat buttermilk:** Take 2¼ cups of thick yoghurt and add ¾ cup of water. Now whisk it well using a wooden whisk or electric hand blender until the butter separates. Remove the cream completely and drink the buttermilk. This is beneficial if you have Kapha disorders like obesity, diabetes and other metabolic problems and if your appetite, digestion and body strength are low.

EAT ACCORDING TO YOUR BODY TYPE

2. **Half-fat buttermilk:** It is prepared in the same way as no-fat buttermilk, but here half of the creamy portion is retained for consumption. You can use it for Pitta imbalances like thirst, burning sensation in the stomach, etc., and when the appetite, digestion and body strength are moderate.
3. **Full-fat buttermilk:** Whisk 2¼ cups of thick yoghurt without adding water and consume this whole. It is recommended for consumption if you have Vata imbalances like dryness in the body, constipation, etc., and if your appetite, digestion and body strength are good.

The Benefits of Buttermilk

- 1 cup of buttermilk + ¼ tsp rock salt powder → Balances Vata dosha
- 1 cup of buttermilk + 1 tbsp of cane sugar powder → Balances Pitta dosha
- 1 cup of buttermilk + powders of black pepper, dry ginger and cumin (¼ tsp each) → Balances Kapha and improves digestion as well

SPROUTS

You can make sprouts with grains, legumes or seeds. Sprouts are nutrient-rich and are not very difficult to make at home. They have a nutty flavour and are crunchy.

- Commonly used grains for sprouting are whole-grain wheat, rye, barley, millet, rice, corn, buckwheat and quinoa.
- Sprouts can also be made from the following legumes: chickpea, dried green peas, lima beans, adzuki beans, kidney beans, soya beans, pinto beans, pigeon pea, mung beans, coral lentils and black lentils.
- Flaxseed, sesame, sunflower, chia, fenugreek, mustard, clover and alfalfa seeds are also used for sprouting.

How to Make Sprouts

Hygiene is very important for making sprouts at home. Use a glass jar or a steel bowl to make sprouts. Find an airy and dark spot in which to place the vessel with the sprouts. Avoid direct sunlight.

- Place the grains/beans/seeds that you are going to sprout in a glass jar or steel bowl. Wash and soak in water overnight (8–12 hours). Use grains to water in the ratio 1:3. Cover the mouth of the container using a cotton or muslin cloth and tie it using a thread. Now find an airy but dark spot to place the container. Avoid putting it in the cupboard or refrigerator. The sprouts will grow at room temperature.
- The next day, drain the water from the container by tilting it, without removing the cloth from the mouth of the container.
- Now pour one glass of fresh water into the container and shake it gently to rinse the grains/beans/seeds. Then discard the water and place the container inside a bowl with the mouth facing down, or at a slanted position so that the grains/beans/seeds come into contact with the wet muslin cloth tied to the mouth of the container.
- Repeat the rinsing and draining processes 1–2 times during the day.
- If the weather is very hot, then you may need to rinse and drain the sprouts 2–3 times.
- It is easy to make sprouts in spring or in the winter, and they are also good for health in these seasons. You will notice tiny sprouts within 3 days. The sprouts are ready to consume when small shoots are visible. However, you can continue rinsing and draining the small sprouts for another 2–3 days or until the sprouts grow to around 3 inches in length.
- Once the sprouts have reached the desired length, rinse them with water, drain well and consume them immediately or refrigerate. If you are refrigerating sprouts, pat them dry using a kitchen towel to remove excess moisture and then transfer them to a covered container and refrigerate. Sprouts can be refrigerated for 2–3 days.

How to Consume Sprouts

As raw sprouts are heavy to digest, it is good to sauté or steam cook them before eating. Sprouts require warm, moist or humid conditions to grow—which are ideal for bacterial growth too, which is why sprouts carry a risk of producing food-borne illness if contaminated. Sprouts are rich in protein and have a high content of essential amino acids, but well-cooked sprouts are always preferable to raw ones to maintain healthy digestion.

WATER

It is a general rule that a healthy person has to drink at least 1.5–2 litres of water every day, but it should be adjusted as per one's needs and seasonal changes. Water intake in summer can be about 2–3 litres per day to avoid dehydration, and in winter about 1.5 litres per day is acceptable. If you have a desk job, your water requirement will be less, whereas if you are doing field work, it will be more. Ayurveda prescribes a judicious way of drinking water, which I have summarized below.

Water storage in different vessels and their effects on health are as follows:

Storage Vessel	Effect on Health
Gold	Improves fertility and strength Balances all three doshas
Tin	Increases Kapha
Brass	Enhances immunity Increases Pitta and Vata
Copper	Decreases Kapha Increases Pitta and Vata
Earthen	Balances all three doshas Improves immunity and strength
Iron	Not good

Here are some tips regarding water consumption and its effects on the body:

Water Intake	Effects on the Body
Just before meals	Reduces appetite and leads to emaciation
Immediately after meals	Impairs digestion and leads to weight gain
Large quantities of water or liquid during meals	Weakens digestion
Small quantity of warm or tepid water during meals	Enhances digestion
Cold water	Weakens digestive and metabolic processes
Water stored in a copper vessel	Scraps out excess Kapha and unwanted fat from the body, improves metabolism and helps reduce cellulite

Benefits of Water Energized with Copper

Although drinking water that has been stored overnight in a copper vessel has gained popularity in recent years, its benefits were explained in Ayurveda centuries ago. You can store water in a copper vessel or jug overnight and drink a glass of this water the next morning on an empty stomach, after brushing your teeth. Copper makes the water ionic and helps to maintain the body's acid–alkaline balance. It also has antimicrobial activity.[13] As copper oxidizes naturally, the copper jug/vessel you use to store water has to be washed gently at regular intervals. You may use half a lemon or some freshly squeezed lemon juice mixed with salt or some baking soda mixed with water to rub the vessel, and then rinse the vessel with plain water.

> **Should You Drink Hot Water?**
>
> Hot water is appetizing, easy to digest, good for the throat and helps reduce fat and endotoxins from the body. As water is heavy in coastal regions, it requires rigorous heating. So it is good to boil water and reduce the quantity by half before using it for drinking. In desert-like regions, water is light, so a little heating itself is enough. Water should be boiled and reduced by one-fourth in desert-like regions.

Hot Water	Action on Doshas	Usage According to the Season
Water boiled and reduced by one-fourth	Reduces Vata	Winter
Water boiled and reduced by half	Reduces Pitta	Monsoon, spring, summer
Water boiled and reduced by three-fourth	Reduces Kapha	Autumn

Although water is a nectar necessary for sustaining life, when used in the wrong way (drinking too much at a time, drinking more than what is needed or drinking less than what is required by your body) it may not give you the desired health benefits and can cause health problems like compromised digestive function, low appetite, etc. So be mindful about drinking the correct quantity of water throughout the day.

10

COOKING PRE-PREP

'Cooking is an art, but all art requires knowing something about the techniques and materials.'

—Nathan Myhrvold

Roasted Cumin Seeds

- Heat a heavy skillet over a medium flame. Add 1 cup of cumin seeds and dry roast them for about 7–10 minutes until they are fragrant, smoking and the colour of the seeds changes to dark brown. Stir occasionally to prevent the cumin seeds from being burnt.
- Remove from the fire and when the seeds cool down, you may grind them to a coarse powder using a spice grinder or the pulse mode of a mixer-grinder. Then transfer it to an airtight container.
- This stays good for up to 3 months. You can add ¼ tsp of this roasted cumin seed powder to a cup of buttermilk or have it directly after a meal to enhance digestion.

Roasted Peppercorns

- Roast 1 cup of peppercorns in the same way as the cumin seeds but only for 3–5 minutes. Roasting the peppercorns makes them less hot.
- You can use whole roasted peppercorns or grind them to a coarse powder in a mixer-grinder.

- Although they can be stored in an airtight container for up to 3 months, use freshly roasted peppercorns for the most intense flavour. They add a smoky flavour to dishes and pair well with grilled vegetables. You can sprinkle them over roasted potatoes, use them as salad dressings or simply add them to soups.
- The flavour of peppercorns can diminish during cooking, so it is best to use them towards the end of cooking.

Roasted Asafoetida

- In ¼ cup of ghee, add 1 cup of asafoetida powder and fry over a moderate flame till the asafoetida turns light brown and the pungent smell is gone.
- Transfer it to an airtight container when it has cooled down to room temperature. This stays good for up to 3 months.
- Many people tend to get gas and bloating upon eating lentils or cruciferous vegetables; adding asafoetida to them can help prevent gas and improve digestion. However, as asafoetida has a strong smell and taste and exerts a heating effect on the body, it does not suit everyone. Roasting asafoetida in ghee helps to mellow out the bold smell and taste of asafoetida and reduces the heating effect on the body.

Roasted Turmeric

- In ¼ cup of ghee, add 1 cup of turmeric powder and fry it over a moderate flame till the turmeric turns dark in colour and becomes fragrant.
- Once it cools down, store it in a moisture-free airtight container, away from direct heat and in a dark, cool and dry place. This stays good for up to 3 months at room temperature.
- By frying turmeric in ghee, the flavour is enhanced and the bioavailability of turmeric is increased, allowing the body to absorb and benefit from its healing properties more effectively. This has numerous health benefits and can be added to a variety of dishes,

including soups, curries and stews, and can even be applied as a spread on toast. Or simply add ¼ tsp of this powder to a glass of warm milk or water and enjoy. It helps prevent seasonal allergies and recurrent cold and cough, reduces joint pains, promotes heart health and boosts immunity.[14]

Coconut Milk

- Grate the flesh of a mature coconut using a hand grater. Put the grated coconut in a blender. Add 1 cup of water and blend till the coconut is ground well.
- Strain this into a bowl using a muslin cloth or a cloth strainer. Press the mixture with a ladle to strain all the milk.
- Blend the mixture again, adding 1 cup of water. Strain this mixture into another bowl. This is a thinner milk that is less creamy than the first, but is flavourful and nutritious.
- Depending on the desired consistency and flavour, the thick and thin coconut milk are used in different dishes.
- Coconut milk mellows out the spicy heat in food, creating a more nutty, creamy and balanced flavour.
- Thick coconut milk is used in curries due to its rich flavour and higher fat content, whereas thin coconut milk is suitable for soups and stews where a lighter flavour is desired. Coconut milk is also used in rice dishes and desserts.

RECIPES FOR VATA

1. Ginger Bliss
2. Lemon Splash
3. Mango Delight
4. Tangy Tamarind Juice
5. Citrus Fusion
6. Green Mango Smoothie
7. Coco Bliss
8. Benne Blend
9. Hing Ksheera
10. Vata Latte
11. Gud Ksheera Blend
12. Buttermilk Blend
13. Pomegranate Crush
14. Yoghurt Relish
15. Beet Blend
16. Power Pro
17. Lentil Pesto
18. Garlic Dip
19. Mint–Yoghurt Sauce
20. Berry Dip
21. Mango Salsa
22. Golden Spread
23. Ginger Jam
24. Sweet Millet Bomb

25. Creamy Coconut Milk Porridge
26. Nutri Pancakes
27. High-Protein Flatbread
28. Sweet Flatbread
29. Rice Bread
30. Golden Crisp
31. Veggie Flatbread
32. Savoury Yellow Cake
33. Black Lentil Porridge
34. Peppery Pineapple Soup
35. Quinoa Bowl
36. Zing Rice
37. Lentil Curry
38. Coco–Veggie Gravy
39. Okra Stew
40. Spinach Stir-Fry
41. Mixed Veg
42. Fresh Cheese Balls
43. Ajwain Pudding
44. Lentil Delight
45. Banana Smash
46. Fluffy Froth
47. Rice Pudding
48. Bliss Balls/Bars
49. Milk Lush
50. Sesame Treat

1. Ginger Bliss

This is a perfect drink for winter mornings to keep away cold, cough, aches and pains.

Makes: 1 cup; Preparation time: 10 minutes; Effect on doshas: V- K-*

Ingredients

- 1 tsp cumin seeds
- 1 cup hot water
- 2 pinches dry ginger powder
- 1 tsp honey (optional)
- 1 tsp lemon juice (optional)

Method

- Coarsely grind the cumin seeds using a hand pounder or spice grinder.
- Heat the water in a pan and add the dry ginger and cumin; cover the pan with a lid and allow it to steep for 5–7 minutes.
- Filter with a fine mesh strainer and drink it hot/lukewarm.
- You may also add honey (only when the drink is lukewarm) and lemon juice if you wish.

Notes

- To make this easier, you can use a tea infuser to hold the cumin seeds and dry ginger, and when the steeping is done, you can easily remove the infuser from the vessel.
- Other spices/herbs that can be used for making herbal infusions are mentioned in the table below. Use one or more of these in combination.

---

*Increase is indicated as +

Decrease is indicated as −

For example, V+ means it will increase Vata and V- means it will reduce Vata/balance Vata.

Spices	Herbs
Anise	Ashwagandha (*Withania somnifera*)
Caraway	Dashmool (Root of 10 herbs)
Coriander	Bala (*Sida cordifolia*)
Cardamom	Brahmi (*Bacopa monnieri*)

2. Lemon Splash

A refreshing blend to revive, restore and revitalize

Makes: 1 cup; Preparation time: 10 minutes; Effect on doshas: V-

Ingredients

- 1 cup water
- 2 tsp jaggery powder
- 2 pinches dry ginger powder
- ¼ tsp cardamom powder
- ½ slice lemon (seeds removed)

Method

- Heat the water in a pan. Add the jaggery powder and mix well using a spatula to dissolve it uniformly.
- Now filter it through a cloth strainer to remove any debris.
- When the liquid becomes lukewarm, add the dry ginger powder and the cardamom powder.
- Squeeze half a lemon into it. Mix well and enjoy.

3. Mango Delight

Who doesn't love mangoes? Treat yourself with this super delicious, sweet beverage in the summertime.

Makes: 1 cup; Preparation time: 15 minutes; Effect on doshas: V- P+ K+

Ingredients

- 1 cup ripe mango, skin and seed removed, cut into cubes
- ½-inch piece fresh ginger
- ¼ tsp clove powder
- ¼ tsp cardamom powder

Method

- Grind the mango and ginger using a blender or food processor.
- To this, add the remaining ingredients, mix well and serve.

Note

- If you feel it is too concentrated, you may add ¼–½ cup of water to it as per your desired consistency, then mix well and serve.

4. Tangy Tamarind Juice

Enjoy this mouthwatering, tangy, sweet juice that is rich in tartaric acid and great for improved digestion and liver health.

Makes: 1 cup; Preparation time: 15 minutes; Effect on doshas: V- P+ K-

Ingredients

- ¼ cup ripe tamarind fruit, skin and seeds removed
- 1 cup water
- 1 pinch fresh ginger, grated
- 1 pinch black pepper, crushed
- 1 pinch clove powder
- 1 tsp rock sugar
- 1 pinch edible camphor (optional)

Method

- Put the tamarind fruit in a glass or stainless-steel bowl.
- Heat the water in a saucepan and add it to the bowl of tamarind fruits. Now cover the bowl with a lid.
- Allow the tamarind fruit to soak in the water for 10 minutes. This will help to soften the tamarind and make the extraction of the pulp easier.
- Macerate the tamarind fruit in water using your fingers or a masher.
- Filter the tamarind water into a new bowl using a fine mesh strainer and use a spoon to squeeze out as much extract as possible.
- Now add the other ingredients to the filtrate and mix well using a spoon, then serve.
- If you feel the drink has a very strong taste, you may add another ½ cup of water to dilute it. Enjoy this drink at room temperature.

Note

- To make this preparation easier, you may use tamarind paste instead of tamarind fruit. If using tamarind paste, you can add it to lukewarm water and mix it in directly. There will be no need for soaking.

5. Citrus Fusion

A zesty drink with a punch of Vitamin C

Makes: 1 cup; Preparation time: 10 minutes; Effect on doshas: V-

Ingredients

- 1 tsp freshly squeezed citron juice
- 1 tsp rock sugar powder
- 2 pinches black pepper powder
- 2 pinches roasted cumin powder
- 1 cup water
- ½ tsp finely chopped mint leaves (optional)

Method

- In a glass, add 1 tsp of freshly squeezed citron juice. Then add the other ingredients. Mix well using a spoon and serve.

6. Green Mango Smoothie

A hydrating and energizing drink

Makes: 2 cups; Preparation time: 30 minutes; Effect on doshas: V- P+

Ingredients

- 2 cups water
- 1 cup unripe green mango, skin peeled, seed removed, cut into small pieces
- 4 tsp rock sugar powder
- ¼ tsp black pepper powder
- 2–3 pinches clove powder
- 1 pinch edible camphor (optional)

Method

- Heat water in a saucepan and add the chopped mango. Cover and cook on a medium flame for 10 minutes.
- Then remove the lid and pierce one of the pieces of mango with a fork to check if it is soft and well cooked. If it is hard, cook for 5 more minutes on a medium flame without covering it.
- Now switch off the flame and let the mango cool down to room temperature.
- Then blend the mango in a blender to a smooth, edible consistency and transfer it to a glass.
- Add the other ingredients—powders of rock sugar, black pepper, cloves and edible camphor. Mix well and serve.

Note

- Avoid using fibrous mangoes.

7. Coco Bliss

A creamy and delicious coconut drink, this healthy non-dairy buttermilk can reset your metabolism.

Makes: 1 cup; Preparation time: 15 minutes; Effect on doshas: V- K+

Ingredients

- 1 cup tender coconut flesh
- 1 tsp lemon juice
- 1–2 pinches rock salt (optional)

Method

- Add the tender coconut flesh to a blender and blend it well. Transfer it to a glass.
- Now add the lemon juice and salt, mix well and serve.

Note

- You can use coconut milk instead of tender coconut flesh. If using coconut milk, avoid the addition of salt. Whisk the coconut milk and then slowly add lemon juice to it. Mix well and serve.

8. Benne Blend

A gentle nutty-flavoured beverage. Fall in love with this silky-smooth beverage packed with calcium and protein.

Makes: 1 cup; Preparation time: 5 minutes; Effect on doshas: V- K+

Ingredients

- 6 tsp white sesame seeds
- 1 cup milk
- 1 cup water
- 1 tsp honey
- 2 pinches cinnamon powder

Method

- Coarsely grind the sesame seeds in a mixer-grinder.
- In a saucepan, add the coarsely ground sesame seeds, milk and water. Boil this on a moderate flame until the water evaporates, that is, until only 1 cup of liquid remains.
- When it is lukewarm or cools down to room temperature, add the honey and cinnamon powder, then mix well and serve.

9. Hing Ksheera

A strong-tasting potion, this nutritious recipe lubricates your intestines, relieves bloating and softens stools.

Makes: 1 cup; Preparation time: 5 minutes; Effect on doshas: V-

Ingredients

- 1 tsp ghee
- 2 pinches asafoetida powder
- 1 cup skimmed milk
- 2 green cardamom pods, crushed

Method

- In a frying pan, heat the ghee. Add asafoetida powder and sauté for a minute. Keep it aside.

- Heat the milk in a saucepan and add the cardamom pods. When it comes to a boil, lower the flame and add the asafoetida fried in ghee (along with the extra ghee in the frying pan) to it. Continue heating it for 30 seconds while stirring once in a while.
- Remove from the heat. Drink this ksheera when it is lukewarm.

10. Vata Latte

A comforting and warm drink to de-stress your mind and body

Makes: 1 cup; Preparation time: 5 minutes; Effect on doshas: V-

Ingredients

- 1 cup full-fat milk (it is not necessary to remove the cream)
- ¼ tsp green cardamom powder
- 2 pinches nutmeg powder
- ¼ tsp dry ginger powder
- ¼ tsp turmeric powder
- 1 tsp rock candy or jaggery powder or as required (optional)

Method

- Bring the milk to a boil in a saucepan. Add the other ingredients (except the sweetener—rock candy/jaggery powder) and simmer for 1–2 minutes.
- Remove the saucepan from the heat. Add the rock candy or jaggery powder, mix well, then transfer the drink to a cup and consume it hot/warm.

11. Gud Ksheera Blend

A nourishing recipe for lung support

Makes: 1 cup; Preparation time: 5 minutes; Effect on doshas: V- K-

Ingredients

- 1 cup goat milk
- 2 pinches black pepper powder
- 2 pinches turmeric powder
- 1 pinch cinnamon powder
- 2 tsp palm jaggery powder

Method

- Bring the milk to a boil in a pan.
- Then remove from the heat and transfer it to a glass. Add the other ingredients. Mix well and enjoy.

Notes

- If you do not have palm jaggery, you may use honey. However, honey should be added only when the milk is lukewarm.
- Vegans can use oat milk instead of goat's milk.

12. Buttermilk Blend

To maintain a healthy balance of gut microbiota and to promote smooth digestion, enjoy this recipe as a post-lunch drink.

Makes: 1 cup; Preparation time: 10–15 minutes; Effect on doshas: V- K+

Ingredients

- ½ tsp sesame oil or coconut oil
- ½ tsp mustard seeds
- ½ tsp cumin seeds
- 1 pinch asafoetida
- 4–5 curry leaves
- ¼ tsp fresh ginger, grated
- 1 tsp onion, finely chopped

- 1 cup full-fat buttermilk
- Rock salt as per taste

Method

- Heat the oil in a small pan, then add the mustard seeds and cumin seeds.
- When the mustard seeds splutter and the cumin seeds are fried (make sure not to burn them), add the asafoetida.
- Now add the curry leaves, fresh ginger and onion, and sauté for a minute.
- Remove from the heat and add this to the buttermilk.
- Add the salt, mix well and serve.

13. Pomegranate Crush

A wonderful recipe with the sweetness of pomegranate and the richness of yoghurt to prevent digestive disturbances and improve heart health

Makes: ½ cup; Preparation time: 5–10 minutes; Effect on Doshas: V- K+

Ingredients

- 1 cup pomegranate arils
- ¼ cup yoghurt
- 2 pinches cinnamon powder
- 1 pinch clove powder

Method

- Add the pomegranate arils to a blender or food processor. Blend the seeds until the juice is released. Strain the juice through a fine mesh strainer or cheesecloth. Press the pulp using a spoon to extract the juice. Discard the seeds.
- In a separate bowl, churn the yoghurt using a hand blender.

- Add the pomegranate juice, cinnamon and clove powder and mix well. Enjoy.

Note

- Don't blend the seeds too much, or the juice will taste bitter.

14. Yoghurt Relish

A nutritious combination that gives you a feeling of fullness and satiety, which helps to curb cravings

Makes: 1 cup; Preparation time: 5 minutes; Effect on doshas: V-

Ingredients

- 1 cup sweet yoghurt
- 6 tsp jaggery powder, or as per taste
- 2 pinches nutmeg powder
- 1 tsp chia seeds (soaked overnight in water)
- 1 tsp pumpkin seeds

Method

- Add yoghurt and the other ingredients to a bowl and whisk well until well blended. Serve.

Notes

- Use chia seeds along with the water used for soaking.
- If you prefer a low-fat option, you can use buttermilk instead of yoghurt.

15. Beet Blend

Tender beets topped with yoghurt and spices replenish energy levels and make for a refreshing drink

Makes: 1 cup; Preparation time: 10 minutes; Effect on doshas: V-

Ingredients

- 1 cup yoghurt
- ¼ cup sweet beets, grated
- ¼ tsp black pepper powder
- ¼ tsp clove powder
- ¼ tsp salt, or as per taste

Method

- In a bowl, add the yoghurt and whisk it. Now add the sweet beets, black pepper and clove powders and salt to the yoghurt, mix well using a spoon and serve.

Note

- You can use grated carrots or finely chopped mangoes instead of sweet beets in the recipe.

16. Power Pro

A power drink for all ages to boost your energy and mood

Makes: 75 servings; Preparation time: 45–50 minutes; Effect on doshas: V- P-

Ingredients

- ¼ cup sorghum
- ½ cup pearl millet
- ½ cup finger millet
- ¼ cup mung lentil (preferably without skin)
- ¼ cup wholewheat grains
- 6 tsp red rice/whole rice
- 6 tsp sago

- 6 tsp horse gram
- ¼ cup foxtail millet
- 7–8 almonds
- 6–7 cashews
- 1 tsp cardamom powder
- 1 tsp dry ginger powder

Method

Prepare the mixture:

- You can dry roast each ingredient one by one in the same skillet or combine some ingredients that have similar roasting times and dry roast them together. Make sure to stir these continuously to prevent burning.
- Dry roast the sorghum until it puffs up, typically around 3–5 minutes.
- Combine the pearl millet, finger millet, mung lentil and foxtail millet (as they have similar roasting times) and dry roast them over medium heat for about 7–10 minutes, stirring frequently until they are fragrant and slightly toasted.
- Combine wheat, rice, sago and horse gram and dry roast them together for 7–10 minutes or until they start to pop.
- Mix the cashews and almonds and dry roast them for 3–5 minutes until the cashews are browned and the almonds have darkened.
- Now switch off the heat and when the skillet is still hot, add the cardamom and ginger powders and dry roast them for 10–20 seconds. Stir frequently to prevent them from burning.
- Mix all the ingredients (except the powders of cardamom and dry ginger) together and let them cool down to room temperature. Then using a mixer-grinder, blend them in small batches to make a fine powder. Once all the ingredients are ground in different batches, put them in a big bowl, then add the powders of cardamom and dry ginger. Mix well and store in an airtight container at room temperature for up to 3 months. Alternatively, this mixture can also be refrigerated.

Prepare the drink:

- Add 2 tsp of this herbal drink mix to a glass of warm milk or water and consume this daily in the morning or evening.

Note

- You can sift the powder mix using a stainless-steel mesh (size 40) to get a uniform particle size.

17. Lentil Pesto

A unique tasting and easy-to-prepare high-protein pesto

Makes: ½ cup; Preparation time: 15 minutes; Effect on doshas: V- K-

Ingredients

- ¼ tsp sesame oil
- ½ cup yellow mung lentils
- ¼ tsp black pepper powder
- 3 garlic cloves, skin peeled, crushed
- 3 tsp grated coconut
- 2 tsp water
- ¼ tsp rock salt, or as per taste

Method

- Heat the oil in a kadai on a low flame. Add the yellow mung lentil and roast for about 7–10 minutes until the lentils turn golden in colour. You have to keep stirring in between so that the lentils don't get burnt.
- Then turn off the heat and add the black pepper powder and continue stirring for a minute. Let it cool down to room temperature. Then grind it in a mixer-grinder along with the garlic, grated coconut and water. It will become a coarse paste.
- Now mix the salt in it and serve with flatbreads or rice.

Note

- This can be stored in the refrigerator for 2–3 days.

18. Garlic Dip

A hot, flavour-packed, absolutely delicious recipe

Makes: ½ cup; Soaking time: Overnight; Preparation time: 5 minutes; Effect on doshas: V- K- P+

Ingredients

- 10 medium-sized cloves of garlic
- 1 cup buttermilk
- 2 pinches black salt
- 2 pinches carom seed powder
- 2 pinches fried asafoetida powder
- 2 pinches rock salt
- 2 pinches dry ginger powder
- 2 pinches black pepper powder
- 2 pinches long pepper powder
- 2 pinches cumin powder

Method

- Remove the skin and sprouted part of each garlic clove. Then wash them in water and soak them in buttermilk overnight to remove the pungency.
- The next day, remove the garlic cloves from the buttermilk and discard the buttermilk.
- Grind the garlic cloves to a fine paste. Add all the other ingredients, mix well and enjoy with rice or use as a salad dressing.

Notes

- This recipe is not good for summer.
- People suffering from acid reflux should avoid this recipe.

19. Mint–Yoghurt Sauce

A very tasty and creamy, yet low-calorie sauce or dip that can be paired with a variety of dishes

Makes: 1½ cups; Preparation time: 10 minutes; Effect on doshas: V-

Ingredients

- 8 tsp full-fat yoghurt
- 1 cup mint leaves, roughly chopped
- ½ cup coriander leaves, roughly chopped
- ¾ cup onion, roughly chopped
- ¼ capsicum, seeds removed, roughly chopped
- 1-inch piece fresh ginger, skin removed, roughly chopped
- 2 garlic cloves (optional)
- ½ tsp roasted cumin powder
- ¼ tsp rock salt, or as per taste

Method

- Grind all the ingredients together in a mixer-grinder to a fine paste.
- Enjoy this all-purpose dipping sauce that goes with just about everything—as a side dish with flatbreads or pancakes or as a dipping sauce for green salads, snacks and appetizers or simply as a spread for sandwiches.

Note

- This can be stored in an airtight container in the refrigerator for 2–3 days.

20. Berry Dip

A fresh and zingy dip made using only a few ingredients

Makes: 1 cup; Preparation time: 5 minutes; Effect on doshas: V-

Ingredients

- 1 cup blueberries/blackberries, seeds removed
- ½ tsp black pepper powder
- ¼ tsp turmeric powder
- ¼ tsp cumin seeds
- ¼ tsp lemon zest
- ¼ tsp salt, or as per taste

Method

- Add all the ingredients to a mixer-grinder and blend to a smooth paste. Serve with flatbreads.

21. Mango Salsa

A simple, quick, tangy and uplifting treat

Makes: 1½ cups; Preparation time: 15 minutes; Effect on doshas: V-

Ingredients

- 2 tsp flaxseeds
- 1 cup raw mango, skin and seed removed, roughly chopped
- ¼ cup water
- ¼ cup jaggery powder
- 1 tsp cumin seeds
- ½ tsp ginger, grated
- 1 tsp black pepper

- ½ tsp rock salt
- 1 tsp sesame oil
- 1 cup yoghurt (optional)

Method

- Dry roast the flaxseeds in a skillet over medium heat for 2–3 minutes. Then transfer to a plate.
- In the same skillet, add the raw mango and water. Cover with a lid and cook on medium heat for 10–12 minutes or until the mango is 90 per cent cooked.
- Remove from the heat and let it cool down to room temperature.
- In a blender, add the mango (with residual water, if any), flaxseeds, jaggery powder, cumin seeds, ginger, black pepper and rock salt. Blend into a fine paste.
- Add the sesame oil, mix well and serve with flatbreads/savoury pancakes/rice. You can mix it with 1 cup of yoghurt and enjoy it as a mango yoghurt salsa too.
- It stays good in the refrigerator for 2 days.

22. Golden Spread

A sweet, immunity-boosting winter delight for people of all ages

Makes: ½ cup; Cooking time: 45 minutes; Drying time: 1 day; Effect on doshas: V- P-

Ingredients

- ½ cup ash gourd, skin peeled, seeds removed, chopped into ½-inch pieces
- 1 cup water
- 2 tsp ghee
- ½ cup rock sugar powder

- ½ tsp long pepper powder
- ½ tsp dry ginger powder
- ½ tsp cumin powder
- 2 pinches coriander powder
- 2 pinches bay leaf powder
- 2 pinches cardamom powder
- 2 pinches black pepper powder
- 2 pinches cinnamon powder
- 1 tsp honey

Method

- Add the ash gourd and water to a kadai, cover and cook for about 20 minutes.
- Then squeeze the ash gourd in a muslin cloth to extract the juice.
- Collect the ash gourd pieces and dry them in sunlight for 5–6 hours. Then cut them into smaller pieces or pierce them multiple times with a fork and fry them in ghee for 5–7 minutes.
- Now add the juice that was collected earlier. Add the rock sugar and cook it. Keep stirring the ash gourd continuously with a ladle to prevent the contents from sticking to the bottom of your cooking vessel. When a semi-solid mass is obtained, stop cooking. This should take approximately 20 minutes.
- Add the long pepper, dry ginger, cumin, coriander, bay leaf, cardamom, black pepper and cinnamon powders while the mixture is still hot. Mix well to get a homogeneous mass.
- When the mixture becomes lukewarm, add the honey and mix well.
- This jam can be stored in a moisture-free airtight container for up to 2 weeks in the refrigerator.
- You can enjoy this jam with flatbreads or simply stir 1 tsp of this jam into a cup of yoghurt or warm milk/water and enjoy it as a beverage.

Notes

- It is not necessary to get a jam with a smooth consistency. As we are not grinding the ash gourd, there could be some small pieces.
- This recipe can be prepared with yam instead of ash gourd. When prepared with yam, the recipe improves your digestive enzymes, regulates bowel movement, promotes good gut bacteria and is K- V-.

23. Ginger Jam

A yummy jam with a perfect sweet–spicy balance that strengthens the respiratory and digestive systems

Makes: 1 cup; Preparation time: 40 minutes; Effect on doshas: K- V-

Ingredients

- 1¼ cups fresh ginger juice
- 1¼ cups jaggery powder
- 3 tsp bay leaf powder
- 3 tsp cardamom powder
- 3 tsp cinnamon powder
- 3 tsp black pepper powder
- 3 tsp long pepper powder
- 3 tsp dry ginger powder
- 3 tsp clove powder
- 3 tsp nutgrass or cumin powder
- 3 tsp bishop's weed powder
- 3 tsp coriander seed powder
- 3 tsp honey

Method

- In a thick-bottomed vessel, mix the fresh ginger juice with the powdered jaggery and heat it over a medium flame. Stir occasionally to prevent it from sticking to the bottom of the vessel.

- When it reaches a semi-solid consistency (this should take about 15 minutes), add all the dry powders, mix well and continue heating on a low flame for another 10–15 minutes until the mixture thickens further.
- Remove from the heat. When the mixture becomes lukewarm, add the honey and mix well.
- Spread on flatbreads or stir into yoghurt or warm water and consume.

Notes

- To get 1¼ cups of juice, you will need approximately 500–750 gm of fresh ginger. Wash and chop the ginger. Then grind it in a mixer-grinder and squeeze through a fine mesh strainer to obtain the juice.
- Once the jam is prepared, it can be stored in a moisture-free airtight container at room temperature for about 10 days and in the refrigerator for up to 1 month.

24. Sweet Millet Bomb

A fantastic guilt-free snack with the flavour of bay leaf

Makes: 15; Preparation time: 30 minutes; Effect on doshas: V-

Ingredients

- ¼ cup water (or as needed)
- ¼ cup jaggery powder
- 1 cup foxtail millet flour
- 6 tsp coconut, grated
- ¼ tsp cardamom powder
- ¼ dry ginger powder
- ¼ cup ghee
- ¼ cup raisins
- 2 cups ripe bananas, peeled, finely chopped
- 15 fresh bay leaves

Method

- Heat water in a saucepan, add the jaggery powder and stir this mixture. When the mixture comes to a boil, remove it from the heat and filter it using a cloth strainer.

- In a bowl, add the foxtail millet flour, grated coconut, cardamom powder, dry ginger powder, ghee, raisins and the bananas and mix well. Then add the jaggery liquid little by little, kneading the mixture to make a dough. The addition of jaggery water should be adjusted to make a soft dough. When you gently press your finger into the dough, it should be slightly tacky, smooth and elastic, but not so sticky that it clings to your hands. The dough should not become pasty or dry. If the dough is pasty, add more flour and if the dough is dry, add more water to adjust the consistency of the dough.

- Now divide the dough into 15 small, elongated ball-sized portions. Take one portion and roll it between your palms to make a cylindrical shape, about 1½ inches long and ½ inch thick. Repeat with the remaining portions.

- Take a fresh bay leaf and place one portion of the dough in the centre on the back side of the leaf and roll it. Now tuck the leaf stem over the cylindrical portion of the dough so it is well sealed. Repeat with the remaining portions.

- Place 7–8 of these on a plate inside a steamer in only one layer and steam for 15–20 minutes. Do not place one layer over the other as then they may not cook properly. Steam them in two batches. Then remove the bay leaf and enjoy.

Note

- If you do not have fresh bay leaves, you can use plantain leaves (cut into small pieces) or dry bay leaves. When you use plantain leaves or dry bay leaves, you can tie the cylinders with a thread. If you do not have any leaves, then you can steam the balls directly without wrapping them. Wrapping with leaves allows the flavour of the leaves to enter the dish and adds to its health benefits.

25. Creamy Coconut Milk Porridge

An immunity-boosting and gut-healing food recommended during cold weather

Makes: 2½ cups; Soaking time: 5–6 hours; Preparation time: 30 minutes; Effect on doshas: V-

Ingredients

- ½ cup steel-cut oats
- ¼ cumin seeds
- 3 garlic pods, crushed
- 1 tsp fenugreek seeds
- 1½ cups water
- 1 cup coconut milk, homemade /tinned (divided into ½ cup + ½ cup)
- ¼ tsp rock salt (optional)

Method

- Wash and soak the oats in water for 5–6 hours or overnight.
- Crush the cumin seeds using a hand pounder.
- In a thick-bottomed vessel, add the oats, crushed garlic pods, fenugreek seeds, 1½ cups of water (you can use the water used for soaking the oats and, if needed, add more to make a total of 1½ cups) and ½ cup coconut milk. Cook on a moderate flame until the oats are well cooked and become soft. This should take about 25 minutes.
- Now add the remaining ½ cup of coconut milk and cook for 2–3 minutes. Then remove the vessel from the heat.
- Add the crushed cumin seeds and salt. Mix well and serve.

Notes

- You can use brown rice or amaranth in this recipe instead of steel-cut oats.

- If you like a soupy consistency, you can add more water.
- This dish should be consumed as soon as it is prepared as it will become thick and sticky once it cools down. Consuming it warm will increase its health benefits, so you should reheat it if you are eating it later.

26. Nutri Pancakes

A high-protein, nutty flavoured healthy breakfast treat

Makes: 5–6; Preparation time: 35 minutes; Cooking time: 20 minutes; Effect on doshas: V- K-

Ingredients
- 2 cups yoghurt
- 1 cup semolina
- ½ cup chickpea flour
- ½ tsp rock salt, or as per taste
- 1 cup finely chopped vegetables (mix of onion, capsicum, tomato, cabbage, carrot)
- 2 tsp coriander leaves, finely chopped
- 6 tsp sesame oil or ghee (for cooking)

Method

Prepare the batter:

- Add the yoghurt to a bowl and blend using a hand blender.
- Mix the semolina and chickpea flour in another bowl. Add the salt and yoghurt to it. Whisk to create an airy batter without any lumps.
- Cover with a lid and leave it aside for about 20 minutes.

Make the pancakes:

- Check if the batter has a moderate consistency. If the batter is thick, add a little water and mix well.
- Now add the chopped vegetables and coriander leaves and mix the batter using a ladle.
- Preheat a skillet. When it becomes hot, pour one ladle of the batter into the skillet and spread it in a circular motion using the ladle.
- Spread 1 tsp of sesame oil or ghee on the surface of the pancake and along the sides. Cover with a lid and cook over a moderate flame for 2 minutes until golden brown on the bottom and half cooked on the top.
- Flip the pancake with the help of a spatula. Once flipped, do not cover it with the lid. Do press the pancake using the spatula to cook it evenly.
- After 1–2 minutes, when both sides are cooked, remove to a plate and serve with a spread or yoghurt.

Notes

- You can use water instead of yoghurt in this recipe.
- You can refrigerate the batter for up to 2 days. When you want to prepare the pancakes, take the batter out of the refrigerator 30 minutes before you want to make them.
- You can also grate cottage cheese and add it as a topping on the cooked pancakes.

27. High-Protein Flatbread

A lightly spiced savoury flatbread with an extra boost of protein and fibre from sprouted mung

Makes: 3–4; Preparation time: 30 minutes; Cooking time: 15–20 minutes; Effect on doshas: V- K-

Ingredients

- ¼ cup yoghurt
- ¼ cup sprouted mung
- 2 tsp sprouted fenugreek
- ½ tsp ginger, grated
- ½ tsp bishop's weed
- 2 tsp coriander leaves, finely chopped
- ¾ tsp cumin powder
- ½ tsp turmeric powder
- ¼ rock salt, or as per taste
- ½ cup wheat flour
- 4 tsp sesame oil (divided into 1 tsp + 3 tsp)
- Chickpea flour or wholewheat flour, for dusting

Method

Prepare the dough:

- Add the yoghurt and sprouted mung and fenugreek to a mixer-grinder and grind them to a smooth texture. (To know about how to make sprouted mung and fenugreek, please check the sprouts section on Pgs. 63–65).
- Now add the grated ginger, bishop's weed, coriander leaves, cumin powder, turmeric powder and salt to the mixer-grinder and mix well.
- In a wide-mouthed vessel, add wheat flour and the blended yoghurt–mung–fenugreek mixture. Mix well and knead using a spatula or knead the dough with your hands for 5–7 minutes.
- Pour 1 tsp of sesame oil on your palm and knead for a minute to make a big ball. This step helps to remove the sticky dough from your hands, and later when you remove a piece of dough to roll it out, it will not stick to your hands. The dough should be soft. If required (that is, if the mixture is too dry), you may add a little water to make the dough softer.

- Cover the dough with a lid or a wet cloth and leave it for about 20 minutes.

Make the flatbread:
- Now take a golf-ball-sized portion of the dough and roll it between your palms to make a smooth ball. Repeat with the rest of the dough.
- Take 1 ball and flatten it using your palm. Then sprinkle some wholewheat flour or chickpea flour on both sides of the flattened portion.
- Heat a skillet on medium-high heat. While the skillet is getting hot, start rolling the dough into a flat circle using a rolling platform and a rolling pin.
- Roll it gently with even pressure as the thickness should be even. Also, you do not want the flatbread to be too thin because it will become crispy when cooked and won't taste good. You may dust your rolling surface with more flour so the dough does not stick to the rolling platform or the rolling pin. Then flip it and roll it gently on the other side too.
- Once rolled evenly, place it on the hot skillet and maintain moderate heat. In 2–3 minutes, you will see small bubbles appearing on the surface. This means the underside is half cooked.
- Now apply sesame oil to grease the surface of the dough and flip it using a spatula or tongs to cook the other side. The flatbread will puff. Apply sesame oil on this side too and press the centre and edges gently so that it cooks evenly. Cook until golden to dark brown spots appear on the surface. Then remove the flatbread from the skillet and place it on a plate.
- Repeat with the other dough balls and keep stacking them on a plate or keep them in a casserole. If you are storing them in a casserole, place a thick, dry cotton cloth or butter paper in the casserole first and then place the flatbreads on it and cover them with a cloth/butter paper again before you close the lid. Serve hot with yoghurt or a spread.

Notes

- Kneading the dough with your hands for 5–7 minutes makes the flatbreads soft.
- Make sure the flatbreads are cooked properly on both sides. If you think your flatbread is not cooked well on both sides, you can flip it one more time. However, do not flip it too many times as it may become hard and improperly cooked.

28. Sweet Flatbread

A gluten-free flatbread recipe that makes for an energizing breakfast option

Makes: 4–5; Soaking time: Overnight; Preparation time: 30 minutes; Cooking time: 20 minutes; Effect on doshas: V- K-

Ingredients

- 32–35 almonds
- 1 cup finger millet flour + more for dusting
- ¼ cup coconut, grated
- ¼ cup jaggery powder
- ¼ tsp cardamom powder
- 6 tsp ghee (divided into 1 tsp + 5 tsp)
- ½ cup warm cow's milk

Method

Prepare the dough:

- Soak almonds in water overnight. Next morning, discard the water, then peel and remove the skin of the almonds.
- Grind the peeled almonds in a mixer-grinder to make a fine paste.
- Add the finger millet flour to a bowl, then add the ground almond paste, grated coconut, jaggery powder, cardamom powder and 1 tsp

of the ghee and mix well. Now add the warm milk little by little and knead the mixture to make a dough. The dough should be soft and smooth. It should not be too hard or too soft. When you press the dough with a finger, it should make a pit. Now cover the dough using a wet cloth or a lid and keep aside for 20 minutes.

Make the flatbreads:

- Divide the dough into 5 equal portions. Roll each portion between your palms to make a smooth ball.
- Heat a skillet or griddle on a moderate flame.
- Meanwhile, take 1 dough ball, dust a little millet flour on it and place it on a rolling board. Now roll it gently using the rolling pin to make a moderately thin disc. Do not roll it too thin as it may break. Do not roll it too thick as then it may not cook properly.
- Gently place the rolled disc on the hot skillet. When you see bubbles or light brown spots arise on the surface, drizzle 1 tsp of ghee on the top and on the sides and gently flip it to cook the other side. Press on the centre and sides gently to cook the disc evenly. Then drizzle 1 tsp of ghee on this side as well. When brown spots appear on this side, remove it from the skillet and place on a plate.
- Repeat the same with the other dough balls and keep stacking them on a plate or keep them in a casserole.

Notes

- If you feel the proper consistency of the dough is not obtained, adjust the quantity of milk and millet flour.
- You can use almond milk or rice milk instead of cow's milk.
- You can also use coconut oil instead of ghee.
- You can also use wholewheat flour instead of finger millet flour. If using wholewheat flour, this recipe will be extra nourishing and will help a person gain weight.

29. Rice Bread

An easily customizable gluten-free addition to your meal

Makes: 4; Preparation time: 30 minutes; Cooking time: 20 minutes; Effect on doshas: V-

Ingredients

- 2 tsp dill sprigs or basil leaves, finely chopped
- 2 tsp coriander sprigs, finely chopped
- ¼ cup onion, finely chopped
- ¼ cup carrots, skin peeled, grated
- ½ tsp ginger, grated
- 1¼ cup rice flour
- 1 tsp black pepper, crushed
- 1 tsp cumin seeds
- 3 tsp coconut, grated
- ¼ tsp rock salt, or as per taste
- 6 tsp sesame or coconut oil (divided into 1 tsp + 5 tsp)
- ¾ cup water

Method

Prepare the dough:

- Combine all the ingredients (except the oil and water) in a bowl and mix well.
- Then add 1 tsp of oil to it.
- Heat the water in a pan and add it little by little to the ingredients in the bowl while kneading well to make a soft dough.
- Cover it with a lid or a wet cloth and keep it aside for 15–20 minutes.

Make the bread:

- Grease your palms and a plate with oil. Then take one golf-ball-sized portion of the dough and place it on the plate. Gently pat the dough using your palms to flatten it evenly. You can also use butter paper instead of a plate to flatten the dough. The flattened disc should not be too thick or too thin (it should be less than ¼ inch in thickness).
- Now heat a skillet on a medium flame. When it is hot, spread ½ tsp of oil on it. Place the flattened dough on the skillet and cook it on medium flame. After about 2–3 minutes, the base will be a light golden colour. Now drizzle ½ tsp oil on top and the sides and flip it with a spatula to cook the other side. Drizzle ½ tsp oil and cook the bread for another 2–3 minutes or until it becomes a light golden colour. Remove from the heat and place on a plate or in a casserole. Make the rest of the rice breads in the same manner. This versatile bread goes well with dishes ranging from pesto to lentil curry and vegetable gravy.

Note

- You can also soak 3 tsp of pigeon peas in water for 30 minutes, then grind them and add them along with the other ingredients to prepare the rice bread. This will add protein to the recipe.

30. Golden Crisp

A deep-fried yet healthy recipe that is crispy on the outside and soft on the inside but slightly heavy to digest, these tasty golden crisps are best enjoyed by people with a good digestion.

Makes: 4–5; Preparation time: 30 minutes; Cooking time: 20 minutes; Effect on doshas: V- K+

Ingredients

- ¼ cup black lentil flour

- ¾ cup wholewheat flour
- 3 tsp semolina
- ½ tsp coriander seeds, crushed
- ½ tsp fennel seeds, crushed
- ¼ tsp cumin seeds, crushed
- ¼ tsp black peppercorns, crushed
- ¼ tsp dried fenugreek leaves
- ¼ tsp rock salt, or as per taste
- ¼ tsp ginger paste/grated ginger
- 1 pinch asafoetida
- ½–¾ cup water
- 1 cup sesame oil

Method

Prepare the dough:

- In a bowl, add all the ingredients (except the water and oil) and mix well. Then add the water little by little while mixing well to make a dough that is neither soft nor hard. When the dough is prepared, cover it with a lid or wet cloth and leave it aside for 15–20 minutes.

Make the bread:

- Take a lemon-sized portion of the dough and smoothen it by rolling it between your palms. Place it on a round rolling platform or a round plate, drizzle some oil on the rolling area and roll the dough evenly from the centre into a thin disc, using a rolling pin to flatten it. It should not be too thick or too thin—about 0.5 cm in thickness. If it is too thick it won't get cooked properly and if it is too thin, it will become hard when cooked.
- Then heat the oil in a deep pan or kadai on medium heat and when the oil is hot, carefully slide the rolled piece into the oil. When it rises to the surface, gently press it down using a perforated ladle. It will

puff up well. Then flip it carefully and fry the other side as well. This fried lentil bread will be light golden to dark golden in colour when fried properly. Remove it from the oil and place it in a steel colander so that the excess oil is drained out. Fry the rest of the dough balls.

Notes

- After rolling the dough into thin discs, if you do not get proper circles, you can cut the dough using a round bowl of suitable width for perfect circles.
- When cooking, you may check the heat of the oil in the pan or kadai by dropping a small portion of dough into the pan. If the dough rises without browning, that means the oil is hot enough. If it browns quickly, then the oil is too hot, so reduce the flame to allow the temperature to come down. If it stays at the bottom and does not rise up, that means the oil is not hot enough. So wait for the oil to become hot before you start frying. Frying in oil that is not hot enough or when the flame is low will make the dish absorb too much oil. It is important for the oil to be at the right temperature.

31. Veggie Flatbread

Dig into these simple, satisfying and warming flatbreads that are packed with beetroot, herbs and spices.

Makes: 5; Preparation time: 30 minutes; Cooking time: 20 minutes; Effect on doshas: V-

Ingredients

- 1 cup wholewheat flour + more for dusting
- ¼ tsp rock salt, or as per taste
- 4 tsp sesame oil (divided into 1 tsp + 3 tsp)
- ¾ cup beetroot, grated
- ½ tsp ginger, grated

- ½ tsp garlic, grated
- ¼ tsp bishop's weed
- ¼ tsp turmeric powder
- 2 tsp coriander leaves, finely chopped
- ½ cup warm water, or as needed

Method

Prepare the dough:

- Take 1 cup of wholewheat flour in a bowl. Add salt and 1 tsp of oil to it. Combine well. Now add warm water little by little and knead to a soft dough. The dough should not be too tight or too sticky/pasty. Cover the dough with a lid or a wet cloth and keep it aside for 20 minutes. Meanwhile, prepare the stuffing. In another bowl, combine the grated beetroot, ginger, garlic, bishop's weed, turmeric powder, coriander leaves and mix well using a spoon.

Make the flatbread:

- Divide the prepared dough into 5 portions and gently roll each portion between your palms to smoothen it.
- Take 1 ball and place it on the rolling board. Now roll it into a thick disc. Alternatively, you can make a thick disc by placing the dough on the palm of one hand and patting it into shape using the other hand.
- Place 2 tsp of the stuffing in the centre and bring the edges together and seal it.
- Dust some flour on the rolling board. Place the stuffed dough ball on it and roll it gently using a rolling pin to make moderately thick discs. Roll it gently to make sure the stuffing does not come out.
- Heat a skillet on a medium flame. Place the rolled disc in the hot skillet. Drizzle 1 tsp oil on the top and sides. When you see bubbles or light brown spots arise on the top surface, gently flip it to cook the other side. Drizzle 1 tsp of oil on this side as well. When brown

spots appear on this side, remove the flatbread from the skillet and place it on a plate.
- Make the rest of the flatbreads and stack them on a plate or keep them in a casserole. Serve with chutney or yoghurt.

Notes
- You can use carrots or cauliflower or cottage cheese instead of beetroot.
- You can use mint leaves instead of coriander leaves.
- Instead of stuffing the flatbread, you may mix the stuffing ingredients with the wheat flour and make the dough. Then cook them in the same way as the High-Protein Flatbread recipe on Pg. 97.

32. Savoury Yellow Cake

A soft, delicious, healthy and protein-rich rice cake

Makes: 6 cakes; Soaking time: 30 minutes; Resting time: 1 hour; Cooking time: 20 minutes; Effect on doshas: V-

Ingredients
- 1 cup yellow mung
- ¼ cup yoghurt
- ½ tsp cumin seeds
- 1 pinch asafoetida
- ¼ tsp turmeric powder
- 1-inch piece ginger
- ½ tsp rock salt (optional)
- 2 tsp coriander leaves, finely chopped
- Ghee or sesame oil for greasing

Method

- Soak the yellow mung in 2 cups of water for 2 hours. Then drain the water.
- Add the yoghurt, cumin seeds, asafoetida, turmeric and ginger to the soaked mung. Grind this mixture to a fine paste using a mixer-grinder.
- Then transfer it to a bowl, cover it with a lid and keep aside for 1 hour.
- Now add the rock salt, if using, and the finely chopped coriander leaves. Mix well.
- The batter should have a thick and flowing consistency. If the batter is too thick, add a little water to adjust the consistency. If the batter is watery, add a little semolina (about 1–2 tsp or as needed), mix well, cover and leave it for 10 minutes.
- Prepare the cooking equipment (idli steamer or Instant Pot or pressure cooker) in which you are going to place the idli stand. Add 1–2 cups of water to the equipment based on its capacity (the level of water should be just below the first mould of the idli stand) and let the water boil.
- Now grease the idli moulds of the idli stand using ghee or sesame oil and pour 2–4 tsp of the batter (as per the capacity) in each idli mould. Place the idli stand inside the equipment and cover with a lid that has a steam vent. If using a pressure cooker, remove the whistle of the pressure cooker and place the lid tightly on the cooker. Cook for 12–15 minutes on a moderate flame. You can use the steam option in the Instant Pot to cook the idlis.
- Then turn off the stove and let the equipment sit for 5 minutes. Open the lid and check if the idlis are done by inserting a bamboo skewer or a fork into them. If the fork comes out clean, the idlis are ready. If it does not come out clean, cover with the lid and cook for another 3–5 minutes. Once cooked, remove the idlis using a spoon. Serve hot with chutney or a lentil curry.

Note

- You can also make crepes with this batter.

33. Black Lentil Porridge

This super easy, hassle-free and protein-rich recipe is best for those who are looking to increase muscle mass and improve body strength.

Makes: 3 cups; Soaking time: 5–6 hours; Preparation time: 20 minutes; Effect on doshas: V- K+

Ingredients

- ¼ cup black lentils (with skin)
- 1 cup red rice
- 1 tsp fresh ginger, grated
- ½ tsp rock salt, or as per taste
- 2½ cups water
- 1 tsp ghee
- 2 pinches asafoetida
- 1 tsp cumin seeds
- 5–6 curry leaves
- 3 tsp coconut, grated

Method

- Wash and soak the black lentils and red rice in water for 5–6 hours or overnight. Then discard the water.
- In a pressure cooker, add the rice, black lentils, fresh ginger, rock salt and water. Cook on a moderate flame for 5–6 whistles.
- When the pressure is released, open the lid of the cooker.
- Heat a pan on a moderate flame, add the ghee and when it is hot, add the asafoetida, cumin seeds and curry leaves. After 30 seconds, add this to the cooked rice and black lentils.
- Now add the grated coconut and salt. Enjoy warm.

Note

- You can also cook this dish in an Instant Pot or in an open vessel instead of a pressure cooker. If using an Instant Pot or open vessel, the cooking time will be longer and the water required will be more, say 3–3½ cups.

34. Peppery Pineapple Soup

A sweet, spicy, tangy soup with the goodness of pineapple, lentils, herbs and spices for winter or monsoon

Makes: 2½ cups; Soaking time: 30 minutes; Preparation time: 30 minutes; Effect on doshas: V-

Ingredients

To roast and grind

- ¼ tsp pigeon peas
- ¾ tsp coriander seeds
- ¼ tsp split chickpeas
- 1 dry red chilli
- ¼ tsp fenugreek seeds

To make the soup

- ½ cup pigeon peas
- ¼ cup pineapple, skin removed, roughly chopped
- 3 garlic cloves
- ½ tsp cumin seeds
- ½ tsp peppercorns
- 2 cups water (divided into 1½ cups + ½ cup)
- 1 tsp sesame oil
- 2 pinches asafoetida

- ¼ tsp turmeric powder
- 2 tsp coriander leaves, finely chopped
- ¼ tsp rock salt, or as per taste

Method

Roast and grind:

- Heat a pan and dry roast all the ingredients specified under 'To roast and grind' on a low flame for 15 minutes, stirring all the while until the ingredients emit an aroma. Transfer them to a plate and let the mixture cool down to room temperature. Then grind this mixture using a mixer-grinder to get a fine powder.

Prepare the soup ingredients:

- Wash and soak the pigeon peas in water for 30 minutes. Then discard the water.
- Grind the pineapple pieces in a mixer-grinder and filter it using a stainless-steel strainer to get pineapple juice.
- Remove the skin of the garlic and using a hand pounder, crush the garlic cloves, cumin seeds and peppercorns together.

Prepare the soup:

- Cook the pigeon peas with 1½ cups of water in a pressure cooker for 2–3 whistles.
- When the pressure goes off, open the lid and add the crushed garlic mixture, turmeric powder and ½ cup water. Let it boil on a low flame for about 7–10 minutes. Do not cover with a lid.
- Heat the oil in a pan, add the asafoetida and sauté for 2–3 minutes. Then add it to the cooker.
- Remove the cooker from the heat and add the pineapple juice, salt and coriander leaves. Mix well and enjoy.

Note

- You can also add orange juice instead of pineapple juice. However, make sure to add the juice only after removing the soup from the heat as adding it while cooking will make the soup taste bitter.

35. Quinoa Bowl

A mushy quinoa yoghurt recipe for a healthy gut

Makes: 4 cups; Soaking time: 30 minutes; Preparation time: 10 minutes; Cooking time: 20 minutes; Effect on doshas: V- P-K+

Ingredients

- 1 cup red quinoa
- ½ cup yoghurt
- 1¾ cups water
- ¼ cup cucumber, finely chopped
- ¼ cup carrots, finely chopped
- 2 tsp coriander leaves, finely chopped
- 1 tsp sesame oil
- 2 pinches asafoetida
- 1 tsp mustard seeds
- ½ tsp cumin seeds
- 1 tsp ginger, grated
- ¼ tsp rock salt, or as per taste

Method

- Wash and soak the quinoa in water for 30 minutes. Then discard the water.
- Whisk the yoghurt and keep it aside.
- Add the quinoa and water to a saucepan and cook for 20 minutes on a moderate flame. Then remove from the heat and transfer the cooked quinoa to a bowl.

- After 5 minutes, add the whisked yoghurt, salt, chopped cucumber, carrots and coriander leaves. Mix well and keep aside.
- Heat sesame oil in a pan and add asafoetida, mustard seeds and cumin seeds.
- When the mustard seeds pop, add the grated ginger and sauté for a minute.
- Add this mixture to the quinoa. Mix well and serve.

36. Zing Rice

An easy and customizable wholesome meal made with grains, vegetables, aromatics and other ingredients that can be relished with a lentil curry or yoghurt dip

Makes: 2 cups; Soaking time: 30 minutes; Preparation time: 15 minutes; Effect on doshas: V- P- K+

Ingredients
- ½ cup rice
- 2 tsp ghee
- 3–4 almonds, chopped lengthwise
- 3–4 cashews, cut into halves
- 3–4 pecans, chopped into 2 pieces
- 1 seedless date, finely chopped
- 1 apricot, finely chopped
- ½ tsp mustard seeds
- ¾ tsp cumin seeds
- 2 pieces star anise
- 1 bay leaf
- ¼-inch piece fresh ginger, finely chopped
- ¼ cup green peas
- ½ cup vegetables, chopped into ½-inch square pieces (mix of any of these—onion, carrot, sweet beets, zucchini/snake gourd)

- ¼ cup spinach (or lettuce), chopped (optional)
- 1 tsp pumpkin seeds
- ½ cup water
- ½ cup coconut milk
- ½ tsp salt, or as per taste
- 4–5 basil leaves, finely chopped
- 2–3 sprigs coriander, finely chopped

Method

- Wash and soak the rice in 1 cup of water for 30 minutes before cooking. Then discard the water before cooking.
- In a pressure cooker or a thick-bottomed vessel, add the ghee and when it gets hot, roast the nuts and dry fruits and keep them aside.
- Now in the same ghee, add the mustard seeds. When they splutter, add the cumin seeds, star anise and bay leaf and sauté for a minute.
- Then add the fresh ginger, green peas, chopped vegetables and spinach/lettuce and sauté them for another minute.
- Add the rice and pumpkin seeds and sauté for a minute.
- Now add the water, coconut milk and salt and cook this for 2–3 whistles in a pressure cooker or 20–25 minutes in an open vessel. If using an open vessel, add an extra ¼ cup of water.
- Garnish with basil, coriander, roasted nuts and dry fruits and serve with chutney.

Notes

- If you are a vegan, you may use sesame oil instead of ghee. If you are not adding juicy vegetables like zucchini, you may add an additional ¼ cup water.
- You can replace rice with other grains like amaranth or quinoa. If using quinoa, wash and soak for 30 minutes. If you are using amaranth, soak it in water overnight.

37. Lentil Curry

Being rich in dietary fibres and protein, this recipe strengthens your muscles, improves energy and boosts immunity.

Makes: 2 cups; Soaking time: 30 minutes; Cooking time: 25 minutes; Effect on doshas: V- K-

Ingredients
- ½ cup pigeon peas
- 1½ cups water
- ¼ tsp turmeric powder
- ½ tsp garlic, skin peeled, finely chopped
- ½ tsp ginger, skin peeled, finely chopped
- ¼ cup onion, finely chopped
- ½ cup tomatoes, finely chopped
- 1 tsp capsicum, finely chopped
- 2 tsp ghee
- ¼ tsp mustard seeds
- 1 tsp dried fenugreek leaves
- 2 tsp coriander leaves, finely chopped
- 1 sprig of curry leaves
- 2 pinches asafoetida
- ½ tsp rock salt, or as per taste
- 1 tsp cumin seeds

Method
- Wash and soak the pigeon peas in one cup of water for 30 minutes. Then discard the water. Now cook the pigeon peas in pressure cooker along with 1½ cups water for 3–4 whistles. If using an open vessel, add an additional cup of water and cook for about 25 minutes. Once

the pressure is released, open the lid and lightly mash the pigeon peas using a ladle. You can add ½–¾ cup of hot water if you want a soupy consistency.

- Heat the ghee in a kadai on moderate heat and add the cumin and mustard seeds.
- When the mustard seeds splutter, add the asafoetida, curry leaves, ginger and garlic and sauté on a medium flame for 30 to 60 seconds, until fragrant.
- Then add the onion and capsicum and fry them until the onions are translucent. This will take about 3–5 minutes.
- Now add the turmeric powder and sauté for another 30 seconds.
- Then add the tomatoes and salt and sauté for 5–7 minutes, until the tomatoes are soft and well cooked. Now add this to the cooked pigeon peas and simmer for about 5 minutes.
- Then add the dried fenugreek leaves and coriander leaves. Turn off the heat and serve hot with flatbreads or rice.

38. Coco–Veggie Gravy

A sumptuous pot of curry made with coconut paste, yoghurt and a medley of fresh vegetables

Makes: 4 cups; Preparation time: 30 minutes; Effect on doshas: V- P- K+

Ingredients

- 6 tsp yoghurt
- 1 cup coconut, grated
- ½ tsp cumin seeds
- ½ cup water
- 1 yam, skin peeled, chopped lengthwise into 2-inch pieces
- ½ cup raw banana, skin peeled, chopped lengthwise into 2-inch pieces

- 1 drumstick, chopped lengthwise into 2-inch pieces
- 1 cup cluster beans, chopped lengthwise into 2-inch pieces
- ½ tsp turmeric powder
- ½ salt, or as per taste
- ½ cup carrots, skin peeled, chopped lengthwise into 2-inch pieces
- 1 cup bottle gourd, skin peeled, chopped lengthwise into 2-inch pieces
- 1 tsp coconut oil

Method

- Whisk the yoghurt in a blender.
- Grind the coconut together with the cumin and 1 tsp of water in a mixer-grinder.
- In a pan, add the yam, raw banana, drumstick, cluster beans, turmeric powder, salt and ½ cup water. Cover with a lid and cook for 10–15 minutes or until the vegetables are partially cooked.
- Now add the carrots and the bottle gourd, cover with the lid and cook for 5 more minutes. Make sure not to overcook the vegetables.
- Add the ground coconut paste and cook for 5 minutes. Do not cover with a lid.
- Then add the beaten yoghurt and gently toss the vegetables. Make sure not to mash them. Cook on a low flame for 2–3 minutes.
- Then add the coconut oil and remove the pan from the heat. Serve with rice or flatbreads.

39. Okra Stew

A mouth-watering, tangy and mildly spiced ladies' finger recipe

Makes: 2 cups; Soaking time: 30 minutes; Cooking time: 20 minutes; Effect on doshas: V- P-

Ingredients

- 6 tsp pigeon peas
- ½ cup water
- 1 tsp sesame oil
- ½ tsp cumin seeds
- ¼ cup shallots, finely chopped
- 2 tsp fresh ginger, grated
- ¼ cup tomato, finely chopped
- 1 cup ladies' finger, finely chopped
- Salt as per taste
- ½ tsp turmeric powder
- ½ tsp coriander powder
- 2 tsp coriander leaves, finely chopped

Method

- Wash and soak the pigeon peas in water for 30 minutes. Then discard the water.
- Cook the pigeon peas with ½ cup water in a pressure cooker for 2 whistles.
- Heat oil in a skillet and add the cumin and shallots and sauté for 2 minutes.
- Then add the ginger and tomatoes. Sauté for 2–3 minutes or until the tomatoes are well cooked.
- Now add the ladies' finger and sauté on a medium flame for 5–6 minutes until the pieces are cooked to a soft consistency.
- Now add the salt, turmeric and coriander powders and sauté for a minute.
- Add the cooked pigeon peas along with the water and cook on a low flame for 5 minutes.
- Add the coriander leaves, mix well and serve.

40. Spinach Stir-Fry

A treat for your taste buds, with the freshness of spinach and the aroma of garlic

Makes: 1 cup; Preparation time: 15 minutes; Effect on doshas: V- K-

Ingredients

- 1 tsp sesame oil
- ½ tsp cumin seeds
- 1 tsp garlic, skin peeled, finely chopped
- 2 cups spinach (or kale) leaves, washed, finely chopped
- ¼ tsp rock salt, or as per taste
- ½ tsp black pepper powder
- 1 tsp lemon juice

Method

- Heat the oil in a pan on a moderate flame, and when it is hot, add the cumin seeds.
- After about 30 seconds, add the garlic and chopped spinach and fry for 2–3 minutes. Then cover with a lid and cook on medium heat for about 5 minutes. Remove the lid and add salt. Mix well and fry for 2–3 minutes more without covering with a lid.
- Add the black pepper and lemon juice, toss once and serve.

41. Mixed Veg

A colourful, comforting and customizable recipe that is packed with essential nutrients

Makes: 3 cups; Preparation time: 30–35 minutes; Effect on doshas: V- K-

Ingredients

- 2 medium-sized tomatoes
- ¾ cup coconut, grated
- 2 cups + 4 tsp water
- 2 tsp sesame oil
- 1 green chilli, slit lengthwise into two
- ¼ cup colocasia, skin peeled, cut into ½-inch pieces
- ¼ cup colocasia leaves, cut into ½-inch-long pieces
- 1 cup amaranth leaves and stems, cut into ½-inch-long pieces
- ¼ cup yam, skin peeled, cut into ½-inch pieces
- ¼ unripe green banana, cut into ½-inch pieces
- ¼ cup pumpkin, cut into ½-inch pieces
- ¼ cup ridge gourd, outer thick skin scraped slightly, cut into ½-inch pieces
- ½ cup peanuts
- ½ tsp rock salt, or as per taste
- 1 cup corn kernels
- 1 tsp jaggery powder

Method

- Wash the tomatoes and roast them over a gas flame directly for about 2–3 minutes or steam them in boiling water for 5–7 minutes or until the skin starts to peel off. Then remove the tomatoes from the heat, and when they cool down, peel off the skin and gently wash them in water to remove the skin completely.
- Grind the tomatoes and coconut with 4 tsp water to a paste.
- Heat the sesame oil in a pot. Add the green chillies and sauté them for half a minute.
- Then add the chopped leaves and stems of the colocasia and sauté for 2 minutes.

- Add the chopped vegetables, mix well and sauté for 3–5 minutes.
- Then add the peanuts, water and salt. Cover and cook on a moderate flame for 5–7 minutes.
- Now add the corn kernels and the leaves and stems of the amaranth, mix well, cover and cook for 3–5 minutes more or until the vegetables are soft.
- Remove the lid, add the tomato–coconut paste and cook for 5 minutes.
- Add the jaggery powder, mix well and remove from the heat. This can be served with flatbreads or rice or it can be enjoyed by itself.

Note

- If you do not cook the colacasia leaves well, your throat may get itchy when you eat the dish.

42. Fresh Cheese Balls

Soft and spongy sweet cheese balls that are simply magical

Makes: 12 balls; Cheese making time: 40 minutes; Cheese balls making time: 15 minutes; Effect on doshas: V- P-

Ingredients

To make the cheese

- 1¼ cups full-fat yoghurt
- 5 cups full-fat milk

To make the cheese balls

- 2 tsp ghee + more for greasing
- 1 cup fresh cheese
- ¼ cup rock sugar powder
- ¼ cup cardamom powder

- ¼ cup almonds, finely chopped
- ¼ cup raisins, roughly chopped

Method

Make the cheese:

- Whisk the curd in a bowl and keep aside.
- Heat milk in a pan and bring it to a boil.
- Lower the flame and add the whisked curd to it. Mix it well and keep cooking it on a low flame for 3–5 minutes. The milk will curdle and greenish water (whey) will separate. Strain it using a cheesecloth and transfer the solid portion to a bowl.
- Now add room-temperature water to it and rinse it once to remove any sourness. Strain it again using the same cheesecloth. Hold all the ends of the cheesecloth and twist to squeeze out excess liquid.
- Once all the whey has been separated, remove the solid portion and place it on a flat plate. Then cover it with the same cheesecloth and put a heavy weight over it for at least 30 minutes.
- Then remove the weight and the cheesecloth. Transfer the cheese to a bowl and crumble or grate it.

Note

- You will get approximately 1 cup of cheese. However, the quantity of cheese obtained can vary depending on the quality (fat content) of the milk and yoghurt. If the quantity of cheese obtained is less, adjust the quantity of the other ingredients used to make the cheese balls.

Make the cheese balls:

- Heat the ghee in a pan, add 1 cup of crumbled cheese and the sugar and continue heating the pan on a low flame. Keep stirring to prevent the contents from sticking to the bottom.
- After 5 minutes, remove the pan from the heat.

- Add the cardamom powder, chopped almonds and raisins. Mix well.
- Grease your hands with ghee. Take 2 tsp of the mixture and roll it between your hands to make golf-ball-sized balls. Repeat with the remaining mixture.
- This can be stored in an airtight container in the refrigerator for up to 2 days.

Note

- You can also use regular dairy milk/regular yoghurt instead of full-fat milk/full-fat yoghurt. However, do not use skimmed milk as it is fat-free and will not yield any cheese.

43. Ajwain Pudding

A unique tasting dessert to purify, heal and restore the body, this pudding is also recommended for new mothers after a normal delivery.

Makes: 2 cups; Preparation time: 30 minutes; Effect on doshas: V-

Ingredients

- ½ cup ghee
- 1 cup wholewheat flour
- 1 cup water
- ¼ cup jaggery powder
- ¾ tsp bishop's weed powder
- ¼ tsp dry ginger powder
- 1 pinch cardamom powder
- 2 dried figs, finely chopped
- 2 seedless dates, finely chopped
- 4–5 almonds, finely chopped

Method

- Heat the ghee in a skillet. Add the wholewheat flour and roast on low heat until it is lightly browned and smells nutty. It will also start releasing ghee. This may take 10–12 minutes.
- Meanwhile, heat the water in a pan and add the jaggery powder to it. Keep stirring it at regular intervals. When the jaggery powder is completely dissolved and the solution starts to bubble, remove from the heat and filter it using a cloth filter.
- Add the bishop's weed and dry ginger powders to the wheat flour roasted in ghee. Mix well for 30 seconds.
- Then add the filtered jaggery water to it little by little, stirring the mixture continuously using a spatula to prevent the contents from sticking to the bottom and lumps from forming.
- Cook until the mixture thickens and reaches a pudding-like consistency. This will take about 10–12 minutes.
- Sprinkle cardamom powder over it and garnish with chopped dry fruits and nuts. Serve hot.

Note

- You can prepare the above recipe with finger millet flour instead of wholewheat flour. As finger millet is drying in nature, it is good to add ¼ cup of grated pumpkin (with skin and seeds removed) and 1 tsp of dried melon seeds along with the dry fruits while garnishing. When prepared with finger millet flour, this can be a healthy dessert option to satisfy the sweet cravings of a person looking to lose weight.

44. Lentil Delight

A nutrient-dense recipe offering energy, high protein and micronutrients

Makes: ¾ cup; Soaking time: 8 hours; Cooking time: 35 minutes; Effect on doshas: V- P-

Ingredients

- ¼ cup black lentils (with skin)
- 2 tsp raisins
- ¼ cup cashews, each cut in half
- ¼ cup ghee
- 1¼ cups cow's milk

Method

- Wash and soak the black lentils in water overnight or for about 8–12 hours. Discard the water the next day and double-check to make sure there is no residual water. You may also use a dry cloth to absorb any remaining moisture from the lentils.
- Heat the ghee in a kadai. Now add the cashews and raisins and fry them on medium heat for about 3–5 minutes while stirring frequently. When the cashews turn golden brown and the raisins plump up slightly, remove them from the kadai and keep aside.
- In the same kadai, add the black lentils to the remaining ghee and fry on low heat till they become brownish and aromatic. This will take about 5–7 minutes.
- Now add the milk to it and continue to cook on low heat, stirring at regular intervals, until the lentils are tender and creamy and the milk is slightly thickened. This should take approximately 20–30 minutes.
- Remove from the heat, add the fried cashews and raisins. Serve.

Notes

- If you want to add sweetness, rock sugar can be added to the recipe at the end.
- If you prefer a smooth consistency, you can also blend the mixture using a hand blender.
- You can prepare this recipe using mung lentils instead of black lentils.
- Rice milk or oat milk can be used instead of cow's milk.

45. Banana Smash

This rich, sweet and super smooth dessert is fulfilling for toddlers and adults alike.

Makes: 1 cup; Preparation time: 25 minutes; Effect on doshas: V- P-

Ingredients

- 1 ripe, medium-sized banana
- ¾ cup water
- 1 tsp jaggery powder
- 1 tsp ghee
- ½ cup finger millet flour

Method

- Steam the ripe banana in a steamer for 15 minutes.
- Then remove the skin of the banana and add the steamed fruit to a bowl. Mash it using a ladle or potato masher.
- Boil the water in a saucepan and add the jaggery powder to it. Mix well and strain it using a cloth strainer.
- Heat the ghee in a skillet. Add the finger millet flour and fry it on low heat for about 5 minutes while stirring continuously, until the flour emits a slightly nutty aroma.
- Add the jaggery syrup to it little by little and keep stirring well to prevent any lumps. Cook it for about 5–7 minutes or until the mixture thickens.
- Now add the mashed banana to it, mix well and enjoy.

46. Fluffy Froth

A delectable mid-morning or mid-afternoon delight that is light on the stomach because of the addition of spices and pomegranate.

Makes: 1 cup; Preparation time for hung yoghurt: 2 hours; Preparation time for fluffy froth: 5 minutes; Effect on doshas: V- P-

Ingredients

- 2 cups fresh full-fat yoghurt (not sour)
- ¼ tsp dry ginger powder
- ¼ tsp black pepper powder
- ¼ tsp long pepper powder
- ¼ tsp clove powder
- ½ cup pomegranate arils

Method:

Prepare the yoghurt:

- Take a large bowl and place a strainer over it. Line the strainer with a cheesecloth or a muslin cloth and pour the yoghurt over it. Tie the cloth together and keep the yoghurt wrapped tightly in it for at least 2 hours. You can also leave it overnight. However, if you are leaving it overnight, you can keep the whole apparatus in the refrigerator (if you leave it outside at room temperature, the yoghurt will become sour). It will be better to put a heavy object over the yoghurt bundle. This will help in removing the excess whey.

Make the dish:

- Put the strained yoghurt in a bowl and whip using a whisk or wooden churner for about 1–2 minutes until smooth and fluffy.
- Now add the other ingredients to it and whisk once again but for 30 seconds only. The dish is ready to serve.

Notes

- This dish tastes good when served cold. It will be better to keep it in a clay pot in your kitchen or in an airtight container in the fridge before you eat it. If you refrigerate this dish, it can stay good for up to 3 days. If using a clay pot, it can stay good for up to 24 hours in summer and 48 hours in winter.
- As yoghurt is the main ingredient, to get a good flavour, it should be fresh and not sour. You can use full-fat yoghurt to get more hung yoghurt content than whey.
- If you do not have the time to make hung yoghurt at home, you can also use Greek yoghurt to make the recipe right away.
- You may also add ¼ cup of finely chopped nuts and dry fruits like almonds, pistachios, raisins, seedless dates and ¼ tsp cardamom powder, a pinch of nutmeg powder, 3–4 saffron strands and 6 tsp rock sugar powder along with the other ingredients specified in this recipe.

47. Rice Pudding

A perfectly nutritious recipe to start the day

Makes: 1 cup; Soaking time: Overnight; Cooking time: 30 minutes; Effect on doshas: V- P-

Ingredients

- ¼ cup red rice
- 5–6 almonds
- 2–3 dates
- 5–6 raisins
- 2–3 saffron strands
- 2 tsp + 1½ cups full-fat milk
- 2 tsp ghee

- 6 tsp rock sugar powder
- 1 ripe, medium-sized banana, chopped into ½-inch pieces

Method

- Soak the red rice in 2 cups of water overnight. Then drain the water.
- Soak the almonds, dates and raisins in a cup of hot water for about 10 minutes. Alternatively, you can soak them in water at room temperature overnight. Then drain the water. Peel off the skin of the almonds and slice them lengthwise. Remove the seeds of the dates and slice them lengthwise.
- In a cup, add the saffron strands and pour 2 tsp of milk into it just before cooking.
- Boil the remaining milk in a saucepan and simmer it until it reduces to half its quantity. The milk will get condensed, and a layer of cream will form on the top. Remove the saucepan from the heat and keep it aside.
- Heat a thick-bottomed vessel and add the ghee. When it is hot, add the red rice and stir-fry for 2 minutes.
- Then add the condensed milk along with the creamy layer to the red rice and let it cook on a low flame for about 20 minutes. Stir in between to prevent the red rice from sticking to the bottom of the vessel.
- When the red rice is fully cooked and becomes soft, add the rock sugar, raisins, dates, almonds, banana and the saffron soaked in milk. Mix well and serve.

Note

- You can use buckwheat groats instead of red rice in this recipe. If using buckwheat groats, this recipe will be good for balancing Kapha. Instead of rock sugar powder, one may use honey. However, honey has to be added when the dish is lukewarm and not when it is hot.

48. Bliss Balls/Bars

These energy balls make for a nutritious snack.

Makes: 15; Preparation time: 20 minutes; Effect on doshas: V-

Ingredients

- ½ cup sesame seeds
- ¼ cup ghee
- ½ cup cashew nuts, roughly chopped
- ½ cup almonds, roughly chopped
- ½ cup walnuts, roughly chopped
- ½ cup seedless dates, roughly chopped
- ½ cup raisins, roughly chopped
- ½ cup dried figs, roughly chopped

Method

- Dry roast the sesame seeds in a skillet for 3–5 minutes over medium heat while stirring them occasionally. The seeds will start emitting an aroma. Transfer them to a plate and let them cool down to room temperature.
- In the same skillet, add ghee and heat it. Now add the chopped nuts and dry fruits and roast for 7–10 minutes. Then remove from the heat and let it cool down to room temperature.
- Transfer the roasted sesame seeds, chopped nuts and dry fruits (and the remaining ghee, if any) to a mixer-blender and grind for 10–15 seconds/pulse. (If you grind the mixture for too long, it will become a paste.) Transfer to a plate.
- Roll the mixture into lemon-size balls and store them in an airtight container. This stays good for up to 1 month at room temperature and up to 3 months in the refrigerator. You can consume one ball a day. Kids will just love it.

Notes

- If the mixture is too dry and not rolling into a ball easily, add more dry fruits (chopped/ground) or honey. If the mixture is too sticky, add more nuts (chopped/ground).
- If you are a vegan, you can use coconut oil instead of ghee.
- You can also coat the balls in coconut flakes or oat flour. If you coat them, they will keep well at room temperature for about 10 days and in the fridge for about 15 days.
- You can also mould them into different shapes, like square bars, instead of balls.

49. Milk Lush

This dish nourishes the lungs and improves liver function.

Makes: 3 cups; Preparation time: 45 minutes; Effect on doshas: V- P-

Ingredients

- 4 cups milk
- ½ cup ghee + more for greasing
- 1 cup long pepper powder
- 2 cups rock sugar
- ¼ cup honey
- 1½ tsp cardamom powder
- 1½ tsp cinnamon powder
- 1½ tsp bay leaf powder

Method

- Boil the milk in a saucepan.
- Meanwhile, heat the ghee in a kadai. Add the long pepper powder and fry on a moderate flame for 5–7 minutes until it emits a strong aroma.

- Now add the hot milk little by little while mixing well simultaneously using a spatula, so there are no lumps.
- Then add the rock sugar powder, mix well and cook on low heat until the mixture attains a semi-solid consistency. This will take about 25 minutes.
- Remove from the heat and let it cool down a bit.
- When it is lukewarm, add the honey and cardamom, cinnamon and bay leaf powders. Mix well to produce a homogenous dough-like mass.
- This can be used as a spread or you can simply mix 1 tsp of this paste with warm water and consume it once or twice a day.
- You can store it in an airtight container in the refrigerator for about 5 days.

Note

- If you do not have long pepper, you can replace it with black pepper.

50. Sesame Treat

An extremely simple two-ingredient no-bake dessert for a daily sweet treat during winter

Makes: 5; Preparation time: 20 minutes; Effect on doshas: V- P+

Ingredients

- 1 cup black sesame seeds
- ½ cup jaggery powder
- 2 tsp ghee

Method

- Dry roast the sesame seeds in a skillet over medium heat for about 5–7 minutes, stirring occasionally until they pop, emit a toasty aroma and turn darker. Now transfer them to a bowl.

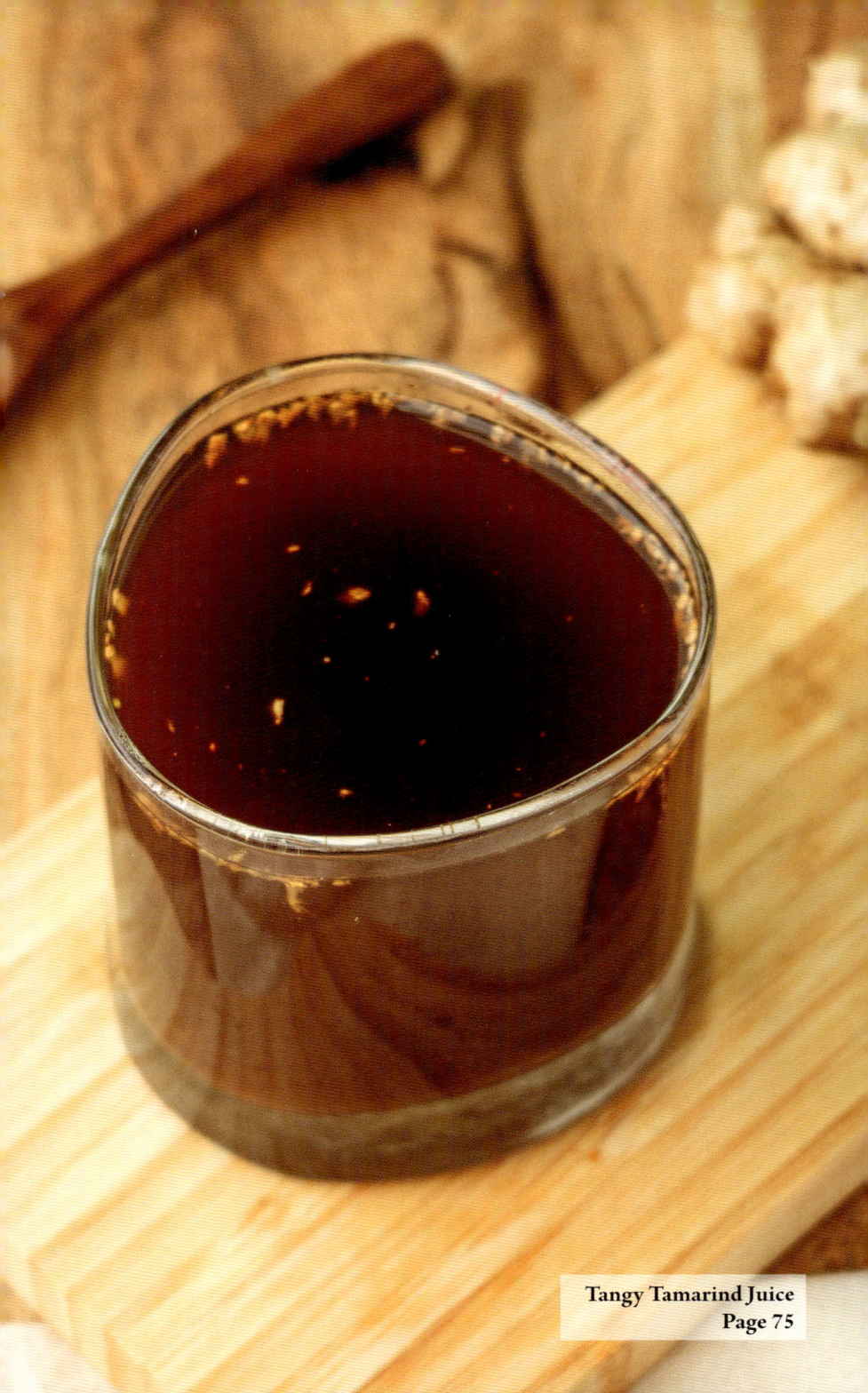

Tangy Tamarind Juice
Page 75

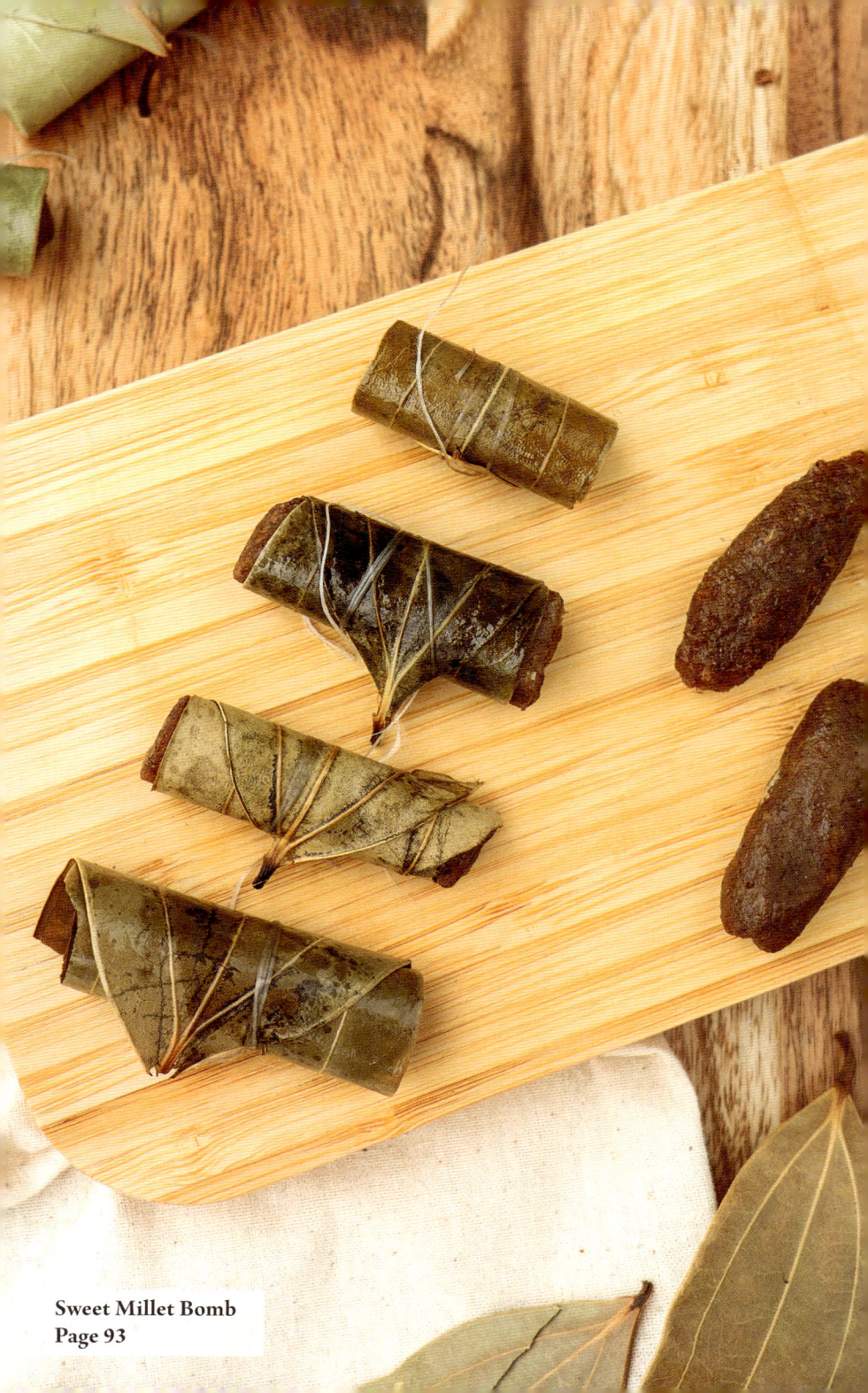

Sweet Millet Bomb
Page 93

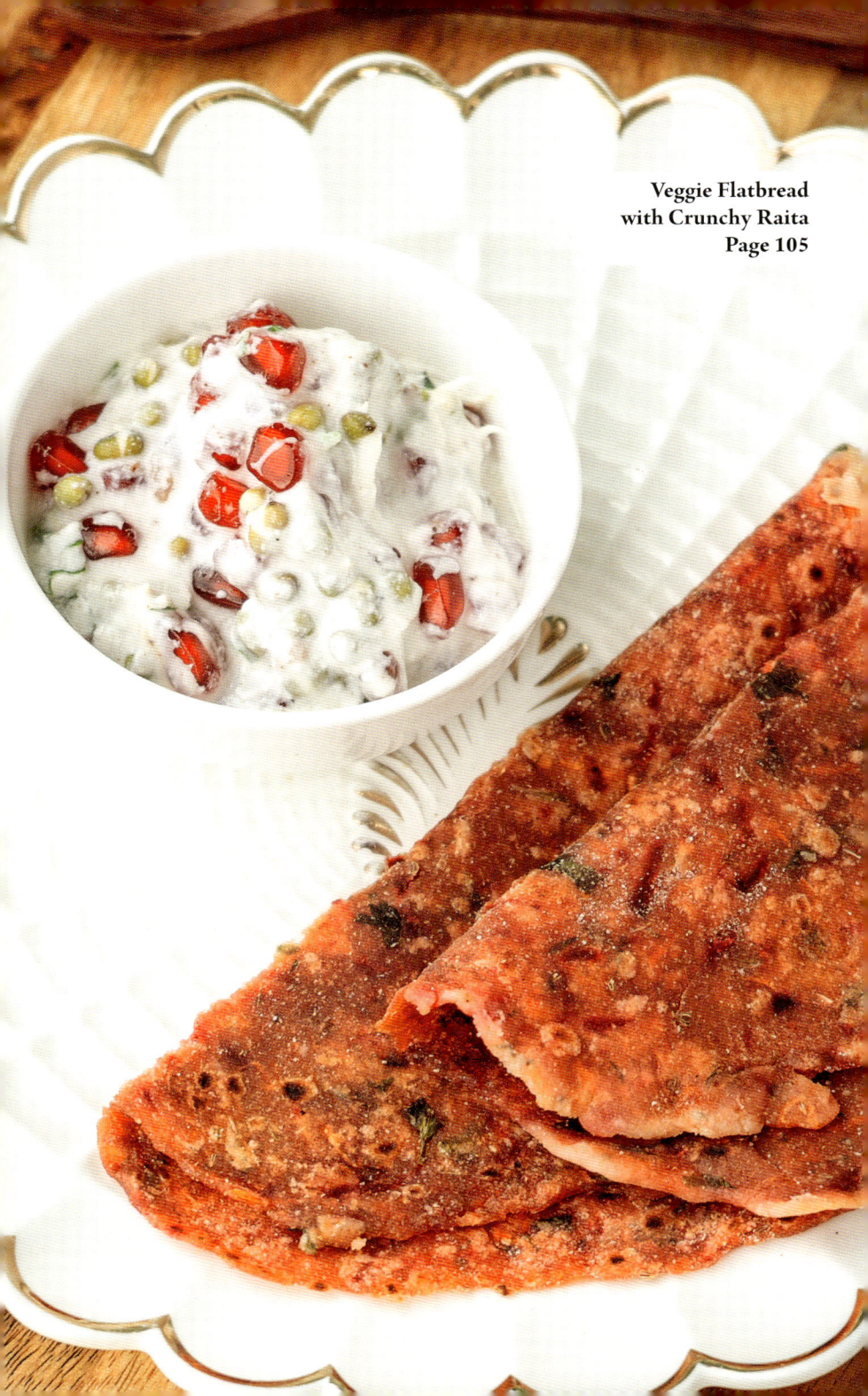

Veggie Flatbread with Crunchy Raita
Page 105

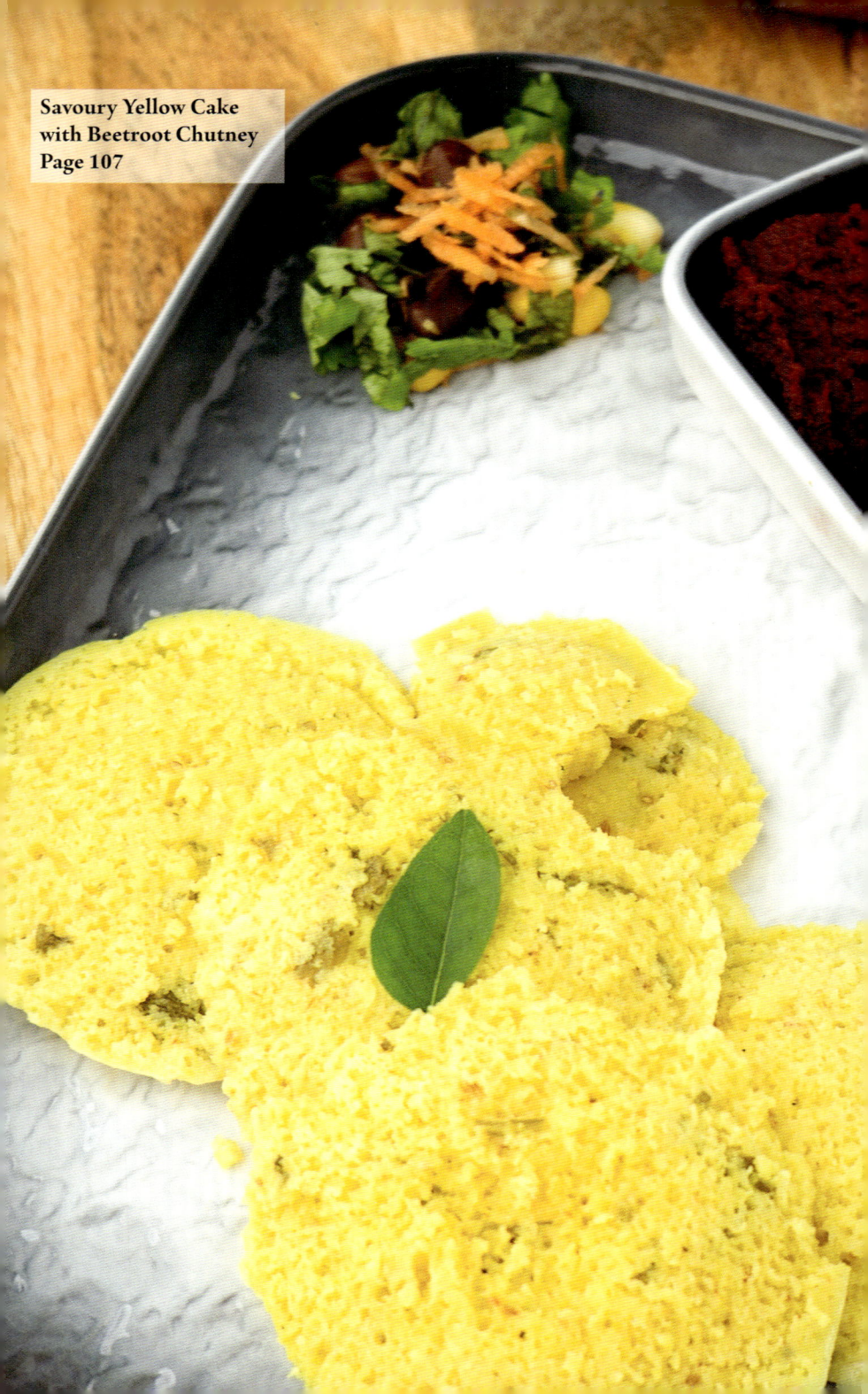

Savoury Yellow Cake with Beetroot Chutney
Page 107

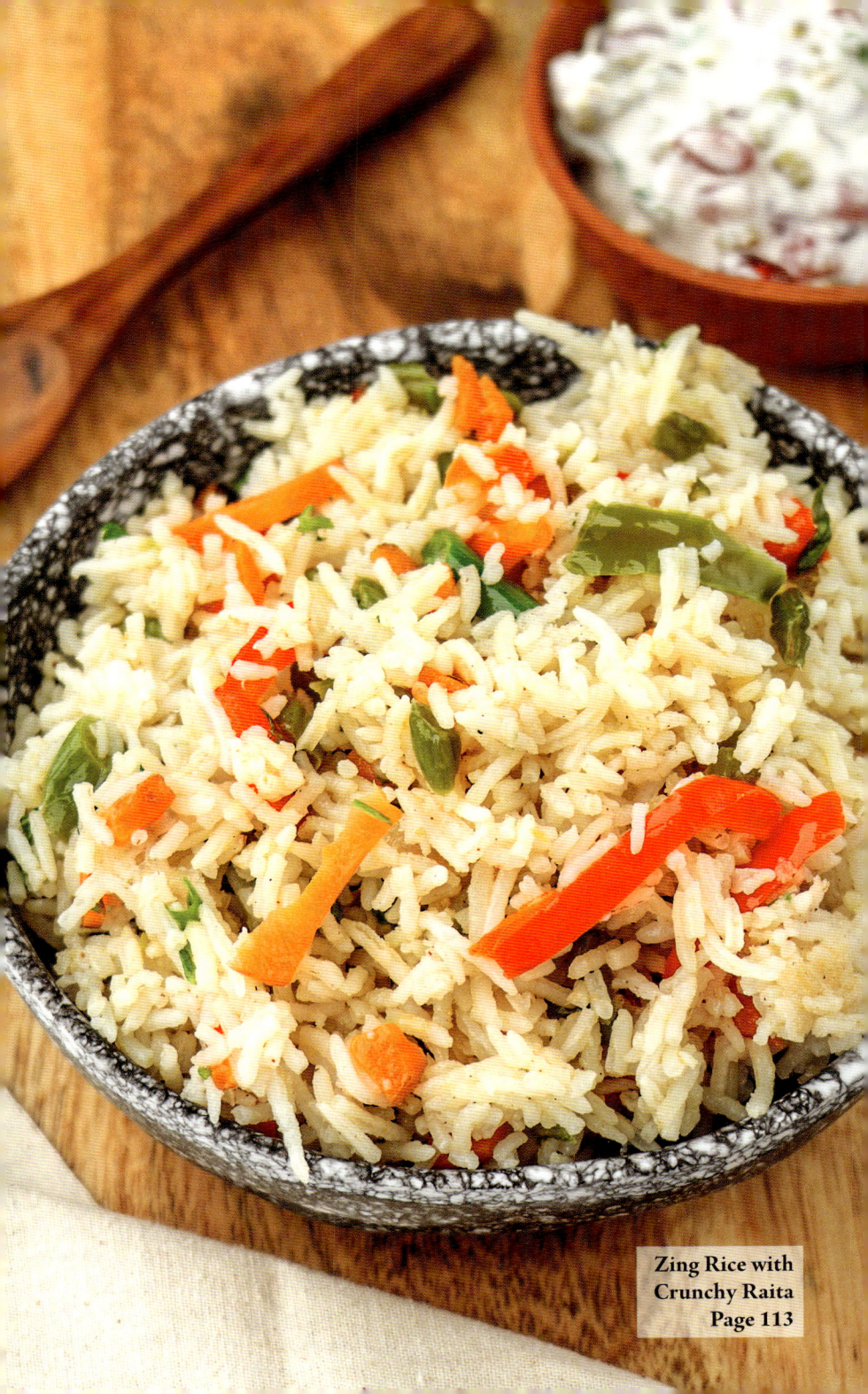

Zing Rice with Crunchy Raita
Page 113

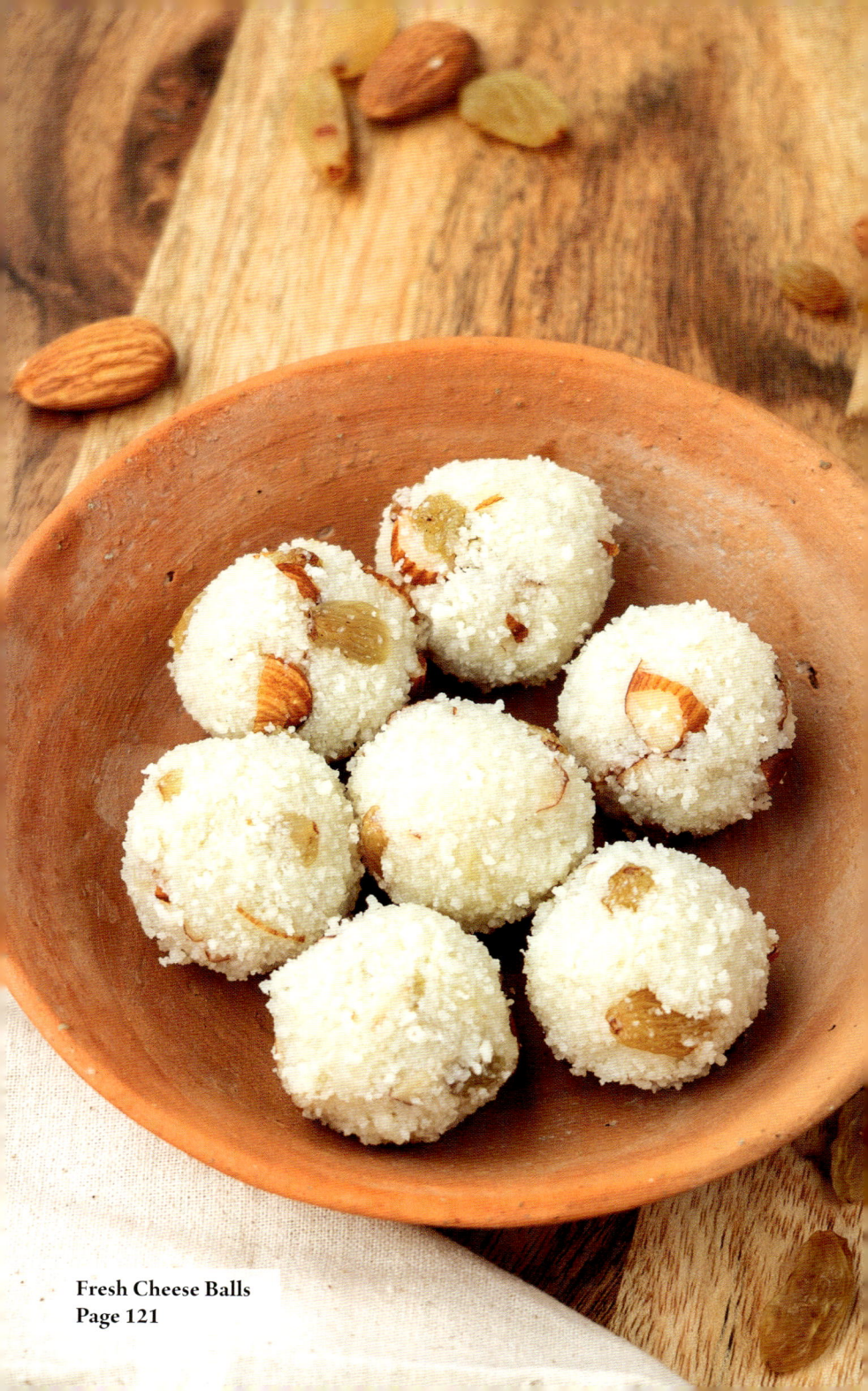

Fresh Cheese Balls
Page 121

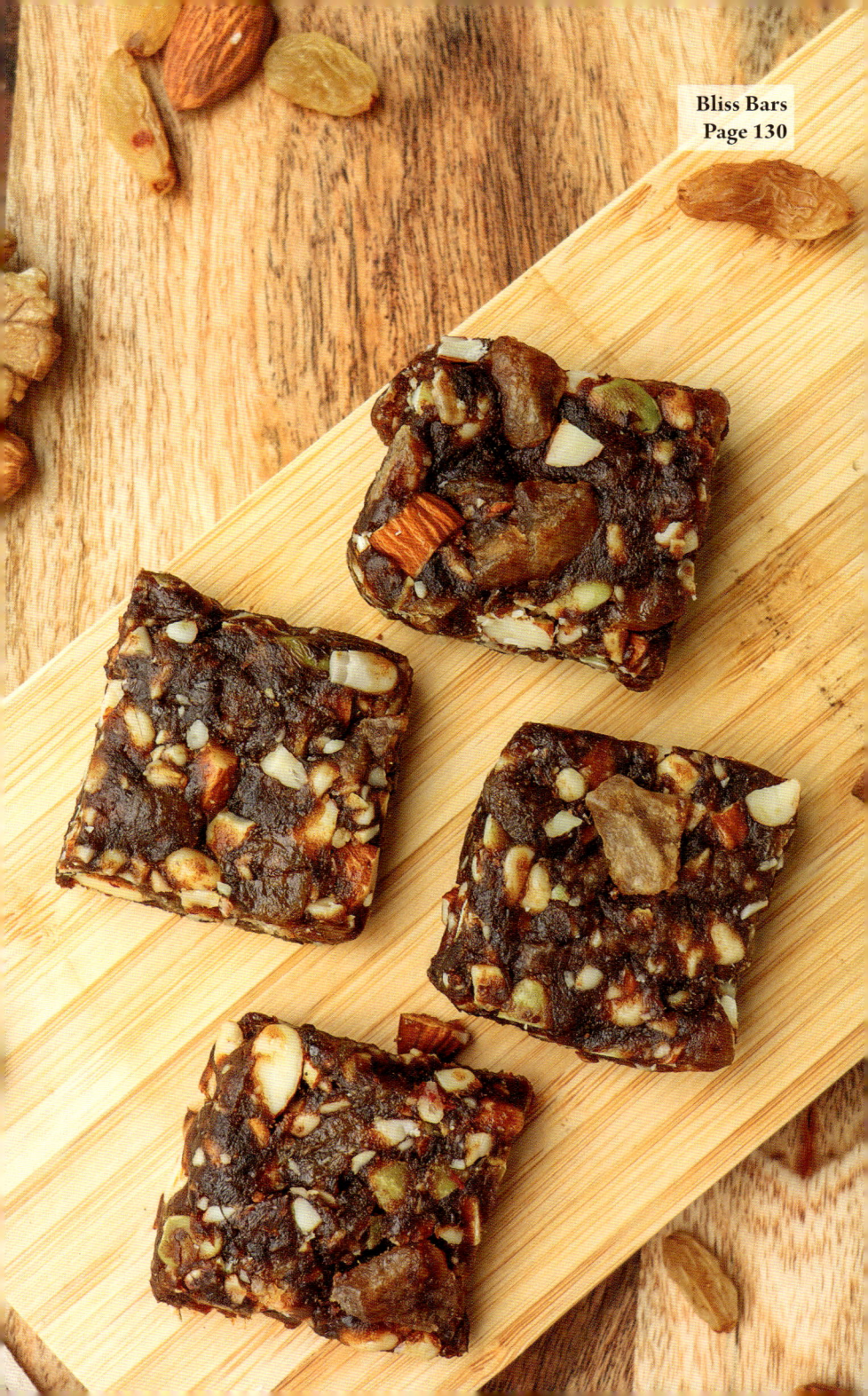

Bliss Bars
Page 130

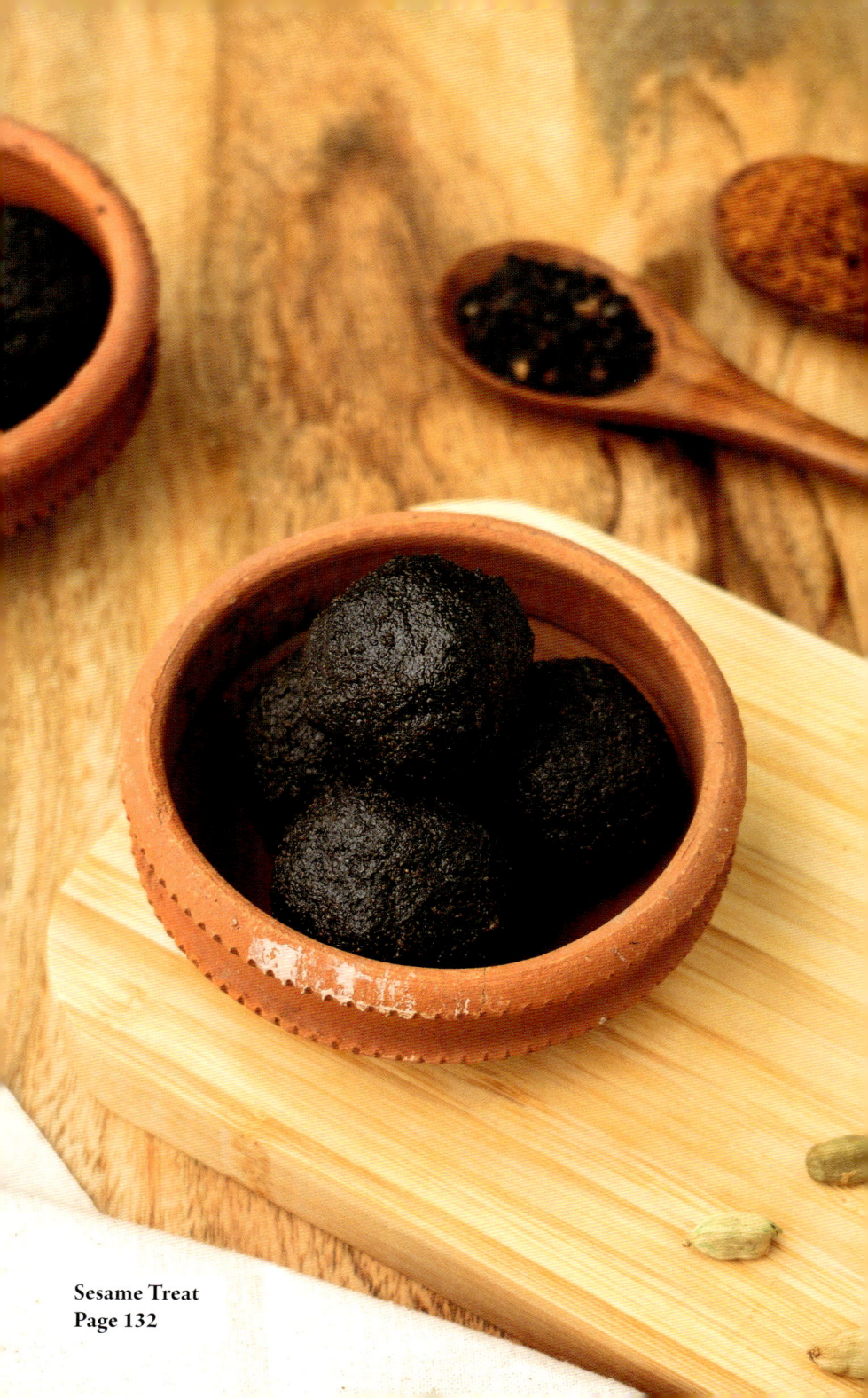

Sesame Treat
Page 132

- Add jaggery powder to the seeds and mix well using a spatula.
- When the mixture is warm, pound it using a mortar and pestle or pulse it in a food processor.
- Grease your palms with ghee. Then take about 2 tsp of this mixture, press and shape it between your hands to make a golf-ball-sized ball. Repeat with the remaining mixture.
- Store the balls in a moisture-free airtight container and leave them at room temperature in cold weather. If the weather is hot, refrigerate them. They stay good for up to 30 days.

Notes

- It is not necessary to pulse grind the mixture if you like a crunchy texture.
- About 2 tsp of ginger powder can be added to the above recipe to improve digestion.
- If the mixture cools down, you will not be able to shape it. So make sure to make the balls when it is warm.
- If you feel the mixture is too coarse or it does not bind well, you may add 2 tsp of warm ghee to it and then shape it.
- Consume only 1–2 balls daily as excess intake may result in indigestion.

RECIPES FOR PITTA

1. Fennel Infusion
2. Coriander Drink
3. Coco–Beet Smoothie
4. Barley Thirst Quencher
5. Natural Electrolyte Drink
6. Banana Smoothie
7. Rice Drink
8. Cucumber Cooler
9. Sweet Creamy Beverage
10. Carrot Ksheera
11. Coco Cool Mix
12. Nutri Mix
13. Coco–Coriander Spread
14. Sesame Butter
15. Creamy Dip
16. Raisins Dip
17. Stuffed Rice Balls
18. Oats Wheat Dumplings
19. Nuts Chaat
20. Mung Patties
21. Mung Pancakes
22. Wholewheat Crepe
23. Savoury Quinoa Cake
24. Fried Wheat Bread

25. Brown Lentils Flatbread
26. Zingy Salad
27. Chickpea Salad
28. Soulful Mung Soup
29. Carrot–Millet Soup
30. Amaranth Veggies
31. Coco–Quinoa Rice
32. Carrot Yoghurt
33. Purple Cabbage Stir-Fry
34. Sautéed Brussels Sprouts
35. Steamed Carrots
36. Spinach Gravy
37. Lentil–Amaranth Curry
38. Pumpkin Curry
39. Mung–Ginger Pudding
40. Mishti Lush
41. Pumpkin–Yoghurt Summer Treat
42. Almond Treat
43. Amaranth Delight
44. Lapsika
45. Coco Ksheera
46. Avocado Bites
47. Coco–Butter Bars
48. Beet Bars
49. Dessert Balls
50. Millet Sweet Balls

1. Fennel Infusion

This sweet infusion can be enjoyed as a replacement for morning tea/coffee or consumed during or after a meal as it helps neutralize stomach acids, soothes the stomach and provides relief from acidity and heartburn.

Makes: 1 cup; Soaking time: Overnight; Preparation time: 5 minutes; Effect on doshas: P-

Ingredients

- 1 tsp fennel seeds
- 1 tsp mint leaves, finely chopped
- 1 cup water
- 1 tsp rock sugar powder (optional)

Method

- Crush the fennel seeds into a coarse powder using a hand pounder.
- Add the fennel seed powder, mint leaves and water to a cup. Cover the cup with a lid and leave it overnight.
- The next morning, mix the contents using a spoon and filter through a muslin cloth.
- Add rock sugar, mix well and consume.

Note

- Soaking the fennel seeds and mint leaves in a clay pot increases the health benefits.

2. Coriander Drink

A natural coolant for summer, this coriander drink helps relieve excess body heat, burning sensations and thirst.

Makes: 1 cup; Soaking time: Overnight; Preparation time: 5 minutes; Effect on doshas: P-

Ingredients

- 1½ tsp coriander seeds
- 1 cup water
- 1 tsp rock sugar powder (optional)

Method

- Crush the coriander seeds into a coarse powder using a hand pounder.
- Add the powder and water to a cup. Cover the cup with a lid and leave it overnight.
- The next morning, mix the contents using a spoon and filter through a muslin cloth.
- Add rock sugar, mix well and consume.

Note

- Other spices/herbs that can be used to make an infusion are mentioned in the table below. Use one or more of these in combination.

Spices	Herbs
Cardamom, Mint, Coriander, Fennel	Shatavari (*Asparagus racemosus*), Anantamool (*Hemidesmus indicus*), Rose/Taruni (*Rosa centifolia*), Liquorice/Yashtimadhu (*Glycyrrhiza glabra*)

3. Coco–Beet Smoothie

A quick and easy delicious drink packed with essential nutrients that stimulate liver function and increase haemoglobin

Makes: 1 cup; Preparation time: 10 minutes; Effect on doshas: P- V-

Ingredients

- ½ cup coconut, grated
- ¼ cup sweet beets, grated
- ¼ cup water

Method

- In a blender, add the grated coconut, sweet beets and water. Grind it for 2–3 minutes. Then squeeze it through a strainer or cheesecloth and serve.

4. Barley Thirst Quencher

A simple, non-carbonated, refreshing morning drink that gives a hearty dose of fibre, minerals and vitamins and improves the efficiency of your intestines to metabolize nutrients.

Makes: 1 cup; Soaking time: 1 hour; Preparation time: 10 minutes; Effect on doshas: P-

Ingredients

- ½ cup barley grains
- 2 tsp ghee
- ¼ tsp roasted cumin powder
- 1 cup water

Method

- Heat a skillet on a moderate flame. Add the barley and dry roast it for 3–5 minutes while stirring frequently. The barley will turn brown in colour. Transfer it into a bowl or a plate. When it cools down to room temperature, grind it into a coarse powder in a mixer-grinder or with a hand pounder.
- Liquify the ghee by heating it slightly in a pan and add it to the roasted barley powder and mix well.

- Transfer it to an earthen pot or a bowl. Add the cumin powder and water and mix well. Cover the vessel with a lid.
- After an hour, mix the contents of the vessel using a ladle and filter before serving.

Notes

- You can add rock sugar or rock salt for taste.
- If you like a tangy flavour, half a lemon can be squeezed into the drink just before consuming.

5. Natural Electrolyte Drink

A replenishing hydration drink without artificial ingredients, excellent when you lose a lot of fluids from heavy exercise or suffer from heatstroke or a stomach bug

Makes: 2 cups; Preparation time: 5 minutes; Effect on doshas: P- V-

Ingredients

- ¼ cup desi khand/rock sugar powder
- 2 cups coconut water
- ½ tsp cardamom powder
- ¼ tsp clove powder
- 1 pinch edible camphor powder (optional)
- ¼ tsp black pepper powder

Method

- Dissolve the sugar in the coconut water.
- Then add the other ingredients, mix well, filter and drink.

Notes

- This drink should be consumed within 2 hours of making it.
- Plain water can be used instead of coconut water.
- You can also use 2 peppermint leaves instead of 2 pinches of edible camphor powder.

6. Banana Smoothie

This easy and delicious banana smoothie, made with just 4 simple ingredients, is a quick breakfast recipe that is packed with protein and fibre. It is a customizable recipe that is kid-friendly too.

Makes: 1 cup; Soaking time: Overnight; Preparation time: 5 minutes; Effect on doshas: P- V- K+

Ingredients

- 1 tsp chia seeds
- 1 ripe banana
- 1 cup milk
- 1 pinch cinnamon powder

Method

- Soak the chia seeds in a little water overnight.
- Peel off the skin of the banana and chop it into small pieces.
- In a blender, add all the ingredients and blend until smooth. Serve.

Notes

- For extra protein, add 1 tsp of chopped almonds.
- You can replace milk with yoghurt.
- For extra fibre, add 1 tsp of roasted flaxseeds.
- If you want the smoothie to be sweeter, add 1 tsp palm sugar or honey.

7. Rice Drink

A nutritious drink with a probiotic effect

Makes: 1 cup; Soaking time: 2–3 hours; Preparation time: 5 minutes; Effect on doshas: P-

Ingredients

- 6 tsp rice
- ½-inch piece cinnamon
- 2 cloves
- 1 cup water

Method

- Wash the rice in water once or twice.
- Now grind the rice along with the cinnamon and cloves into a coarse powder using a hand pounder or a mixer-grinder.
- In an earthen pot or a glass bowl, add the pounded rice mix and 1 cup of water. Cover with a lid and leave it for 2–3 hours.
- Now mix the contents with a hand churner or a ladle. Filter using a muslin cloth and after discarding the solid contents, drink the liquid obtained.

8. Cucumber Cooler

A healthy and refreshing veggie juice that will keep you cool

Makes: 1 cup; Preparation time: 15 minutes; Effect on doshas: P-

Ingredients

- 1½ cups cucumber, skin peeled, roughly chopped
- 3 cups fennel bulb, roughly chopped
- ¼ cup fresh mint leaves, roughly chopped

- ½ a lemon
- 2 tsp rock sugar powder
- 1 cup coconut water

Method

- Add the chopped cucumber, fennel and mint leaves to a blender or a food processor and grind to a smooth consistency.
- Then squeeze it through a strainer or cheesecloth to get juice.
- Squeeze the lemon into a glass and add rock sugar, coconut water and the extracted juice. Mix well and drink.

9. Sweet Creamy Beverage

A nourishing and soothing drink

Makes: 1 cup; Preparation time: 15 minutes; Effect on doshas: P-

Ingredients

- 5–6 almonds
- 2 green cardamom pods
- ½ tsp fennel seeds
- 1 cup full-fat/skimmed milk
- 1 tsp rock sugar powder

Method

- Powder the almonds in a mixer.
- Crush the cardamom pods and fennel seeds using a hand pounder.
- Add the cardamom pods, fennel seeds and milk to a pan and bring it to a boil on a moderate flame. Let it boil for 1–2 minutes.
- Then remove from the heat and filter the milk.
- Add the almond powder and the rock sugar powder. Mix well and consume while it is still warm.

10. Carrot Ksheera

A super-easy-to-make and delicious drink with simple ingredients for a healthy boost of proteins, vitamins and minerals

Makes: 1 cup; Soaking time: Overnight; Preparation time: 20 minutes; Effect on doshas: P-

Ingredients

- 5–6 almonds
- 5–7 raisins
- ½ cup carrot, skin peeled, grated
- 1 cup cow's milk

Method

- Soak the almonds and raisins in water overnight. The next morning, peel the almonds and chop them.
- Heat the milk in a pan and when it comes to a boil, add the grated carrots and chopped almonds and cook for 5 minutes. Remove from the heat and let it cool down to room temperature. Add this to a blender along with the raisins and grind it. Serve.

Note

- You can replace cow's milk with vegan milk.

11. Coco Cool Mix

A nourishing and healing drink that benefits people suffering from acid reflux and heartburn

Makes: 48 servings; Preparation time: 40 minutes; Effect on doshas: P- V- K+

Ingredients

- ½ cup ghee
- 1½ cups coconut, shredded
- 1½ cups rock sugar
- 3 cups coconut water
- ¾ cups dry ginger powder
- ¼ tsp coriander powder
- ¼ tsp long pepper powder
- ¼ tsp cumin powder
- ¼ tsp fennel powder
- 2–3 pinches cardamom powder
- 2–3 pinches cinnamon powder
- 2–3 pinches bay leaf powder

Method

- Heat a kadai. Add the ghee and when it becomes hot, add the grated coconut and roast it on a moderate flame until it turns brown and emits a good aroma. This should take about 10–12 minutes.
- Then add the rock sugar and coconut water, and as the mixture heats, keep stirring in between to prevent the coconut solids from sticking to the bottom.
- The mixture will slowly become semi-solid at first and then attain a solid consistency. At this time, add all the spice powders and mix well. Keep cooking on a moderate flame while stirring the mixture until it attains a dry granule form.
- Remove from the heat and let it cool down to room temperature.
- You can store these granules in a moisture-free airtight container for 15 days at room temperature. If you store it in the refrigerator, it will stay good for up to a month.

- To make the drink, mix 1 tsp of the granules in 1 glass of warm milk of animal or vegetable origin and drink once daily, either in the morning or evening.

12. Nutri Mix

A nutritional supplement for all ages and a promoter of immunity and general wellness, this healing drink is prepared with a blend of grains, nuts, seeds, rock sugar and other healthy ingredients.

Makes: 75 servings; Preparation time: 45 minutes; Effect on doshas: P- V- K+

Ingredients

- 6 tsp melon seeds
- ¼ cup semolina
- ¼ cup coconut, grated
- 1 cup + 3 tsp ghee
- ¼ cup edible gum crystals
- ¼ cup almonds
- 6 tsp groundnuts
- 5–6 seedless dates
- 5–6 pistachios
- 5–6 cashews
- 2 walnuts
- 30–36 raisins
- ¾ cup wholewheat flour
- 2 pinches bishop's weed
- ¾ tsp ginger powder
- ¾ cup rock sugar powder

Method

- Dry roast the melon seeds in a thick-bottomed vessel for 2–3 minutes and then transfer them to a plate and keep aside.
- In the same pan, dry roast the semolina for 7–8 minutes until it turns brown. Transfer it to a plate.
- Dry roast the grated coconut in the same pan until it turns brown.
- Now heat 2 tsp ghee in the same vessel, add the edible gum and cook on a low flame for 4–5 minutes. The edible gum will puff up and look crisp. Remove it and let it cool down to room temperature. Then grind it.
- Add 1 more tsp of ghee to the pan, fry the chopped dry fruits (except the raisins), dates and all the nuts for 2–3 minutes. Remove them from the pan and let them cool to room temperature. Then grind them.
- Now heat 1 tsp of ghee and fry the raisins until they puff up. Then remove and keep aside.
- Heat the remaining ghee in a pan, add the wheat flour and roast it. Keep stirring and let it cook for 15 minutes. When it is cooked and attains a deep brown colour, add the roasted semolina and cook for 4–5 more minutes.
- Then remove the pan from the heat and add the bishop's weed, ginger powder and rock sugar powder to the wheat mixture. Add the rest of the ingredients one by one, mix well and store in an airtight container when it cools down to room temperature.
- It can be stored for 1 month at room temperature and for up to 3 months in the refrigerator.
- To consume this mixture, you can have 1–2 tsp daily, either eating it directly or mixed with a glass of warm milk of animal or vegetable origin.

13. Coco–Coriander Spread

A flavourful, refreshing and versatile spread that is easy to whip up

Makes: ½ cups; Preparation time: 5 minutes; Effect on doshas: P-

Ingredients

- 1 cup coriander leaves, roughly chopped
- 1 cup coconut, grated
- ½-inch piece fresh ginger, peeled, roughly chopped
- 1¼ tsp rock salt, or as per taste

Method

- Grind the coriander leaves, grated coconut and ginger to a fine paste in a mixer-grinder. Add the salt and mix well. Enjoy with sandwiches or flatbreads or use as a dip with a snack.

Notes

- This can be stored in an airtight container in the refrigerator for 2–3 days.
- You can also use sweet beets instead of coriander. Grate the beets and prepare the recipe in the same manner.

14. Sesame Butter

A smooth and silky condiment power-packed with antioxidants

Makes: ¾ cup; Preparation time: 10 minutes; Effect on doshas: P- V-

Ingredients

- ¼ cup sesame seeds
- 6 tsp fresh unsalted butter

Method

- Heat a skillet on a moderate flame and toast the sesame seeds for 3–4 minutes while stirring frequently. When the sesame seeds emit a nutty aroma, remove them from the heat. Let them cool down.
- Now grind the sesame seeds in a food processor for a minute to get a crumbly paste.
- Transfer them to a bowl, add the butter and mix well. Spread it on toast or flatbread, stir it into soup or dip raw veggies in it and enjoy.

15. Creamy Dip

A fresh and flavourful dip that can be used as a salad dressing or spread

Makes: 1 cup; Preparation time: 20 minutes; Effect on doshas: P-

Ingredients

- ½ tsp ghee
- ½ cup avocado, skin peeled, seed removed, chopped
- ½ cup cooked chickpeas
- 1 tsp lemon juice
- ¼ tsp rock salt, or as per taste (optional)

Method

- Heat a pan, add the ghee and toss the avocado pieces in it for 2 minutes.
- Now transfer the cooked chickpeas and the avocado pieces to a mixer-grinder to make a fine paste.
- Add the lemon juice and rock salt. Mix well and serve with flatbreads or rice or simply use as a dip.

Note

- The above recipe can be prepared with blanched spinach or roasted carrots or beets instead of avocado.

16. Raisins Dip

An appetizing dip that is power-packed with vitamins

Makes: 1 cup; Preparation time: 5 minutes; Effect on doshas: P- V-

Ingredients
- 1 cup raisins
- ¼ tsp rock salt, or as per taste
- ½ tsp cardamom powder
- ½ tsp black pepper powder
- ¼ tsp cinnamon powder
- ¼ tsp bishop's weed
- 2 tsp lemon juice

Method
- If the raisins have seeds, remove them. Now grind all the ingredients combined using a hand pounder for 4–5 minutes or pulse in a mixer-grinder for 1–2 minutes to get a smooth paste. This goes well with flatbreads.

Note
- This recipe can be prepared with dates too. When prepared with dates, it balances the Kapha dosha.

17. Stuffed Rice Balls

These delicious steamed dumplings are made with rice flour dough and a yummy coconut and rock sugar filling.

Makes: 8; Preparation time: 30 minutes; Effect on doshas: P- V- K+

Ingredients

- 6 tsp coconut, grated
- 6 tsp rock sugar powder
- 2 tsp ghee
- ¾ cup water
- 2 cups rice flour
- ¼ tsp rock salt, or as per taste

Method

- Mix the grated coconut, rock sugar and ghee in a bowl. Keep it aside.
- Heat the water in a pan.
- In a bowl, add the rice flour and rock salt, then add the hot water little by little while simultaneously kneading it. If the flour sticks to your hands, grease your hands with a little ghee and knead. If the dough becomes too pasty, add a little more rice flour and knead. If the dough is dry, add a little water and knead. Cover with a wet cloth or a lid and keep aside for 15 minutes. Now divide the dough into 8 portions and roll each portion to make a uniform round shape. Flatten one dough ball to make a disc with a 3½-inch diameter and a thickness of ¼ inches. Now place 1 tsp of the coconut mixture in the centre. Seal the edges. If needed you can use ¼ tsp water to seal the edges.
- Now heat an idli steamer and place the stuffed rice balls in it side by side. Do not place one over the other as they will not cook properly. Cover with a lid and steam for 15 minutes until the rice balls are well cooked.
- Transfer them to a plate and serve.

18. Oats Wheat Dumplings

A perfect meal option with the goodness of complex carbs and fibres

Makes: 30; Soaking time: 2 hours; Preparation time: 10 minutes; Resting time: 20 minutes; Cooking time: 20 minutes; Effect on doshas: P- V- K+

Ingredients

- 1 cup steel-cut oats
- ½ cup fresh yoghurt
- 2 tsp coconut oil
- 1 pinch asafoetida
- ½ tsp mustard seeds
- ½ tsp cumin seeds
- 1 tsp ginger, grated
- ½ tsp black pepper, crushed
- 2 tsp cashews, chopped into halves
- ½ cup semolina
- 2 tsp green peas
- ¼ cup carrots, grated
- 6 tsp French beans, finely chopped
- ¼ tsp rock salt, or as per taste
- 2 tsp coriander leaves, finely chopped
- 1 cup + 4–5 tsp water
- 2 tsp ghee

Method

- Wash and soak the steel-cut oats in 2 cups of water for 2 hours. Then drain the water.
- Whisk the yoghurt in a bowl and keep aside.
- Grind the steel-cut oats into a coarse paste using 4–5 tsp water in a mixer-grinder.
- Heat a skillet on a moderate flame, add the coconut oil and when it is hot, add the asafoetida, mustard and cumin seeds. When the mustard seeds splutter, add the ginger, black pepper and cashews and sauté for 2 minutes.

- Now add the semolina and ground oats mixture and sauté for 5–7 minutes or until the mixture turns light brown.
- Now add the green peas, carrots, French beans and salt. Sauté for 2–3 minutes.
- Then add coriander leaves, mix well and remove from the heat.
- When the mixture cools down to room temperature, add the yoghurt and water. Mix well to a smooth consistency without any lumps. It should have a flowing consistency, not too thick and not too runny. Cover with a lid and let it rest for 20 minutes.
- Heat an appe pan on a moderate flame. Grease the appe moulds with ghee and pour 2 tsp of the batter in each mould. Now dribble a little ghee on top of each appe. Cover the appe pan with a lid that has a steam vent. Let it cook for about 5 minutes.
- Then remove the lid and flip the appe using a spoon to cook the other side.
- Cover again and let them cook for 3–4 minutes. Pierce one appe using a fork to see if it is well cooked. If the fork comes out clean, that means the appe is ready. If not, cook for another 2–3 minutes or as required. Then remove the appe and serve hot with pesto.
- Repeat with the remaining batter.

Notes

- You can make idlis instead of appe with this batter.
- You can also use oats in the recipe. If you're using oats, take ¼ cup of oats, grind it to a powder and fry it with the semolina directly.

19. Nuts Chaat

A protein-rich healthy snack you can munch on any time

Makes: 1 cup; Soaking time: 30 minutes; Preparation time: 20 minutes; Effect on doshas: P-

Ingredients

- 1 cup water
- ¼ cup raisins
- ¼ cup almonds
- 3 tsp coriander seeds
- 3 tsp fennel seeds
- ¼ tsp cumin seeds
- ¼ cup pumpkin seeds
- ¼ cup walnuts, chopped
- 2 pinches black pepper powder

Method

- Heat 1 cup of water and add the raisins and almonds to it. Cover and leave it for 30 minutes. Then discard the water and peel the almonds. Place the raisins and almonds on a kitchen towel to dry any excess water.
- Meanwhile, heat a pan and dry roast the coriander, fennel and cumin seeds for 3–5 minutes. Then transfer the seeds to a plate and let them cool down to room temperature. Then crush them using a hand pounder.
- In the same pan, dry roast the pumpkin seeds for about 3 minutes.
- In a bowl, add the peeled almonds, raisins, chopped walnuts, roasted pumpkin seeds, the roasted and crushed spices and black pepper powder. Mix well using a spoon and serve.

Notes

- You can also use coriander and fennel powders, 2 tsp each, instead of the seeds.
- You can store this in an airtight container at room temperature for up to 1 month. While serving, you may also add 3–4 tsp of grated coconut if you wish.

20. Mung Patties

A delicious and healthy savoury dish prepared with mashed mung and spices

Makes: 6; Soaking time: Overnight; Preparation time: 15 minutes; Resting time: 15–20 minutes; Cooking time: 20 minutes; Effect on doshas: P-

Ingredients

- 1 cup mung
- 1 medium-sized potato
- 3 cups water (divided into 1½ cups + 1½ cups)
- ¼ cup coconut, grated
- 2 garlic cloves
- ¼ tsp rock salt
- Oil for shaping
- ¼ cup ghee for frying

Method

- Wash and soak the mung in 2 cups of water overnight. The next morning, discard the water.
- Add the mung to a pressure cooker and add 1½ cups of water. Cover with a lid and cook for 2 whistles. The mung need not be overcooked.
- When the pressure goes off, remove the lid and filter using a strainer. Discard the water.
- Transfer the cooked mung to a plate and let it cool down to room temperature.
- Meanwhile wash and pressure cook the potato in 1½ cups of water for 2 whistles. When the pressure goes away, remove the potato and peel off the skin. Mash the potato.

- Add the grated coconut and garlic to the cooled mung. Grind it to a fine paste in a mixer-grinder. If needed, you may add a little water to grind it.
- Now transfer the mixture to a bowl, add the mashed potato and salt and mix well. Cover the bowl with a lid and let it rest for 15–20 minutes.
- Grease both your hands with oil. Take a golf-ball-sized portion and roll it between your palms. Then flatten it slightly to a thickness of ¾ inch to make a patty. Make 6 patties from the mixture. Grease your hands with oil each time you shape a patty.
- Then heat a skillet, add 2 tsp of ghee and when the ghee is hot, place 3–4 patties side by side on the skillet (based on the capacity of your skillet) and fry on medium heat. When the base becomes golden and crispy, flip the patties gently with a spatula to cook the other side. Cook until this side becomes golden and crisp. If needed, you may flip the patties one or two times more to cook them evenly. Remove and place them on a strainer or paper towel to remove any excess ghee. Cook the remaining patties in the same manner.
- Serve with coriander chutney or yoghurt.

Note

- If the mung–potato mix is too pasty or watery, you may add a little rice flour and mix well before making the patties.

21. Mung Pancakes

A gluten-free, nutrient-dense, simple, soft, fragrant and savoury dish

Makes: 5; Soaking time: Overnight; Preparation time: 25 minutes; Effect on doshas: P-

Ingredients

- 1 tsp chia seeds

- ¼ cup almonds
- 1 cup whole green mung
- ¼ cup water, or as needed
- ¼ tsp rock salt, or as per taste
- 5 tsp ghee

Method

- Soak the chia seeds and almonds separately in ½ cup of water overnight. Then discard the water. Soak the mung in 3 cups of water overnight. Then discard the water. Peel the almonds.
- Grind the mung, almonds and chia seeds with ¼ cup of water to make a fine paste using a mixer-grinder. You can also grind them in batches. Transfer the ground paste to a bowl. Add salt and mix well.
- Adjust the quantity of water to get a flowing consistency.
- Now heat a skillet or griddle and when it is hot, grease the surface with ghee. Then pour one scoop (approximately 30–40 gm) of the batter into the centre of the griddle using a ladle and gently spread the batter into a flatter circle with the ladle or a flat-bottomed cup. Pour 1 tsp of ghee on the top and sides of the pancake. Then cover and cook for about 3 minutes until you see bubbles on the surface.
- Now flip the pancake. Let it cook for 1–2 more minutes till it turns a nice golden-brown colour and becomes crispy. Remove from the griddle, flip again, fold and serve.

Notes

- The batter should have a nice flowing consistency (it should not be runny though) and not very thick. If the batter becomes runny, add some wheat flour and mix well to get a flowing consistency.
- If the griddle is overheated, you will not be able to spread the batter properly, so sprinkle some water to cool the griddle a bit and then pour the batter.

22. Wholewheat Crepe

Quick and perfect eggless fluffy pancakes made using basic pantry items

Makes: 5; Preparation time: 5 minutes; Setting time: 15–20 minutes; Cooking time: 20–25 minutes; Effect on doshas: P- V- K+

Ingredients

- ¼ cup coconut, grated
- ¼ cup powdered jaggery
- 1 cup wholewheat flour
- 1½–1¾ cups milk
- 6 tsp ghee

Method

- Mix the grated coconut and jaggery powder in a bowl and keep aside.
- Add the wheat flour to another bowl. To this, add the milk in parts and mix it well, using a spoon to make a uniform batter without any lumps. It is advisable to use lukewarm milk or milk at room temperature. Avoid cold milk as it will cause more lumps.
- The batter should not be runny; it should have a medium flowing consistency. So, adjust the consistency of the milk accordingly. Now cover and leave the batter to rest for 15–20 minutes.
- Now heat a skillet or griddle and when it is hot, grease the surface with ghee. Then pour one scoop of the batter into the centre of the griddle using a ladle and gently spread the batter into a flatter circle just like in the previous recipe. Pour 1 tsp ghee on the top and sides of the pancake. Cover and cook for about 2–3 minutes until you see bubbles on the surface.
- Now flip the crepe and let it cook for 1–2 minutes. Then flip again and spread 2 tbsp of the coconut–jaggery mix on one half of the crepe. Now fold it, remove from the griddle and serve.

Notes

- If the batter becomes runny, add some more wholewheat flour and mix well to get a flowing consistency.
- You can also use vegan milk or water instead of milk in this recipe.
- You can avoid the coconut and jaggery filling and serve the crepes with honey.
- You can also make a savoury version of this crepe with just 3 ingredients—wholewheat flour, salt and water. Take 1 cup of wholewheat flour, 1¾–2 cups of water and ½ tsp salt. Mix all these ingredients and prepare the crepes in the same way. This savoury version of the crepe goes well with pesto/lentil curry.

23. Savoury Quinoa Cake

A hearty and healthy protein breakfast option that keeps you energized all day long

Makes: 10; Soaking time: 5– 6 hours; Fermentation time: 5–6 hours; Cooking time: 15 minutes; Effect on doshas: P- V-

Ingredients

- 1½ cups quinoa
- 1 cup rice
- 1 cup black lentils
- ½ tsp fenugreek seeds (optional)
- ½ cup pumpkin, roughly chopped
- ¼ tsp rock salt, or as per taste
- ¼ cup oil for greasing

Method

- Rinse and soak the quinoa, rice, black lentils and fenugreek seeds together for 1–2 hours. Then drain the water.

- Grind the quinoa, rice, black lentils and fenugreek in a grinder by adding a little water (or as much as needed) to make a smooth batter. Transfer the batter to a large bowl, add salt and mix well using a ladle. Cover with a lid and leave it for 5–6 hours in summer and 9–10 hours in winter. The batter will ferment and increase in volume. The batter should have a free-flowing consistency—you can adjust the water accordingly to get this consistency.
- Grind the pumpkin to a paste using a hand blender or mixer. Add it to the idli batter and mix well.
- Grease idli moulds with oil. Pour 2 tbsp of batter into each of the moulds. Heat 2 cups of water in your idli steamer or pressure cooker or Instant Pot. When the water boils, place the idli mould in it, cover the pressure cooker with a lid (without the whistle) and cook for 10–15 minutes or until the idlis are well cooked. To check if the idlis are well cooked, pierce them with a bamboo skewer or fork and see if it comes out clean.
- Remove from the heat. Allow them to rest for 5 minutes. Then grease a knife or spoon with oil and slide them through the idlis to remove them from the mould. Place the idlis in a casserole or serve hot.
- Cook the remaining batter in the same way.

Notes

- While grinding the soaked grains, lentils and fenugreek, do not use too much water as it may make the batter very runny. It should not be very thick or thin.
- If the quantity of ingredients for grinding is large, you can grind them in batches.
- If the quantity of batter is a lot and you do not want to use it all at once, you can refrigerate it after fermentation and use it within 1–2 days in the summer and 2–3 days in the winter.
- You can add grated carrots or beets instead of pumpkin paste.
- You can replace the quinoa with finger millet or steel-cut oats.

24. Fried Wheat Bread

A nourishing breakfast or lunch option that increases stability, muscle strength, vigour, vitality, energy and stamina

Makes: 8; Soaking time: 8 hours; Preparation time: 20 minutes; Resting time: 15–20 minutes; Cooking time: 30–40 minutes; Effect on doshas: P- V- K+

Ingredients

- ½ cup pomegranate arils
- ¼ cup skinned black lentils
- ¾ cup water
- 1¾ cups wheat flour
- ¼ tsp rock salt, or as per taste
- ¼ tsp coriander seed powder
- 1 pinch asafoetida
- 1 cup ghee

Method

- Add the pomegranate arils to a blender or food processor. Grind for 20–30 seconds or until the seeds are crushed well. Place a fine mesh strainer on a bowl and filter the juice. Press using a spoon to get as much juice as possible. Discard the pulp.
- Wash the black lentils and soak them in 3 cups of water for 6–8 hours. Then discard the water.
- In a pressure cooker, add the soaked black lentils and ¾ cup of water. Cook it on a moderate flame for 5–6 whistles.
- When it cools down to room temperature, blend it using a blender.
- Add the pomegranate juice to it, mix well and keep aside.
- Then combine the wheat flour, rock salt, coriander seed powder and asafoetida and mix well. Add the soupy black lentils mixed with

the pomegranate juice little by little while kneading well to make a medium-texture dough. If needed, you may add more water to make the dough.

- When the dough is prepared, cover it with a lid or a wet cloth and leave it for 15–20 minutes.
- Heat the ghee in a kadai and prepare the fried wheat bread as explained in the Golden Crisp recipe on Pg. 103. Serve with vegetable curry or pesto.

Notes

- If the dough is sticky/watery, add more wholewheat flour as required to knead it.
- If you have digestive issues, you can use whole mung instead of black lentils and sesame/coconut oil to fry instead of ghee.

25. Brown Lentils Flatbread

A nutrient-dense yet easy-to-digest delicacy

Makes: 8; Soaking time: 30 minutes; Preparation time: 15–20 minutes; Resting time: 20 minutes; Cooking time: 25–30 minutes; Effect on doshas: P- K-

Ingredients

- ¼ cup brown lentils
- ½ cup water
- ½ tsp turmeric powder
- ¼ tsp black pepper powder
- ½ tsp rock salt
- 1½ cups wholewheat flour
- ½ tsp garlic, finely chopped
- ½ tsp cumin seeds
- ¼ cup ghee/sesame oil

Method

- Wash and soak the brown lentils in 1 cup of hot water for 1 hour. Then discard the water.
- Cook the brown lentils in ½ cup of hot water in an open vessel.
- When it is well cooked, add the turmeric, black pepper and salt and mix well.
- When it cools down to room temperature, blend it to a smooth consistency using a hand blender or mixer-grinder.
- Take the wholewheat flour in a bowl and add the garlic, cumin seeds, 1 tsp oil and blended brown lentils. Mix well using a spatula or knead well to make a soft dough. Cover it with a lid or a wet cloth and leave it for 20 minutes. Then make flatbreads as explained in the High-Protein Flatbread recipe on Pg. 97.

Note

- Prepare fresh and consume fresh. Avoid refrigerating the prepared dough.

26. Zingy Salad

Apart from being a good source of energy, this zingy salad also helps regulate cholesterol and blood pressure levels.

Makes: 1 cup; Soaking time: 2–3 hours; Preparation time: 10 minutes; Effect on doshas: P- K-

Ingredients

- ¼ cup yellow mung
- ¼ cup cucumber, peeled, finely chopped
- ¼ cup carrot, peeled, finely chopped
- 1 tsp coriander, finely chopped
- ¼ cup coconut, grated

- 1 tsp coconut oil
- 1 tsp cumin seeds
- ¼ tsp black pepper powder
- ¼ tsp rock salt, or as per taste
- 1 tsp lemon juice

Method

- Wash and soak the yellow mung in hot water for 2–3 hours. Then discard the water.
- In a bowl, add the soaked yellow mung, chopped cucumber, carrots, coriander and grated coconut.
- Heat the oil in a pan and when it is hot, add the cumin seeds. When they are roasted, pour the tempering into the bowl with the mung salad and mix well.
- Add the black pepper powder, salt and lemon juice, mix well and serve.

27. Chickpea Salad

A crunchy vegan salad for a satisfying lunch

Makes: 2 cups; Soaking time: 5–6 hours; Preparation time: 20 minutes; Effect on doshas: P- K-

Ingredients

- ½ cup chickpeas
- 2 cups water
- ¼ cup cranberries
- ¼ cup purple cabbage, finely chopped
- 1 jalapeno, seeds removed, chopped
- 1 tsp fresh ginger, grated
- ¼ tsp garlic powder

- 1 tsp sesame seeds
- 32–35 almonds, finely chopped
- 6–8 basil leaves, finely chopped

Method

- Soak the chickpeas in water for 5–6 hours or overnight. Then discard the water.
- Add the soaked chickpeas and 2 cups of water to a pressure cooker and cook them for about 5 whistles. When the pressure goes off, strain and discard the water. Transfer the chickpeas to a bowl, add the cranberries, purple cabbage, jalapeno, fresh ginger, garlic, sesame seeds, almonds and basil leaves, then mix well and serve.

Notes

- You can replace the garlic powder with fresh garlic cloves. Chop 1 garlic clove and use this instead of ¼ tsp garlic powder.
- Instead of purple cabbage, you can use spinach or broccoli. If you're using spinach or broccoli, you should steam them before adding them to the recipe.

28. Soulful Mung Soup

A warming and healing spiced (but not spicy!) appetizer for all seasons

Makes: 4 cups; Soaking time: 6–8 hours; Preparation time: 30 minutes; Effect on doshas: P- V-

Ingredients

- ½ cup whole mung
- 2 tsp ghee
- ¼ tsp asafoetida (or 6 tsp jaggery powder)
- 1 tsp dry ginger powder

- 1 tsp coriander seeds
- 1 tsp cumin seeds
- ¼ tsp rock salt, or as per taste
- 1½ cups water

Method

- Soak the mung in 2 cups water for 6–8 hours.
- Cook the soaked mung in a pressure cooker with 1½ cups of water for 4 to 5 whistles or in an open vessel for 30 minutes.
- When it cools down to room temperature, drain the water and keep it aside. Grind the mung to a fine paste using a mixer-grinder.
- Heat a kadai, add the ghee to it and when it is hot, add the asafoetida. After 1–2 minutes, add the other spice powders and sauté for about 1 minute. Then add the mung paste and mix well. You may add the water drained after cooking the mung as per your desired consistency. If you want it soupy, add 1 cup water and if you want thicker soup, add ½ cup water. Continue to cook on a low flame for about 5 minutes while stirring in between. Remove from the fire and serve.

Notes

- If you like a sweet soup, use jaggery instead of asafoetida. Dissolve the jaggery powder in the water drained after cooking the mung and use it in the recipe. However, if you're adding jaggery powder, avoid salt.
- You can also use sprouted chickpeas instead of mung in the above recipe. If you're using sprouted chickpeas, you do not have to soak them overnight in water. You can cook them directly in a pressure cooker. Do not add jaggery powder if using sprouted chickpea. Use asafoetida and the other spice powders.

29. Carrot–Millet Soup

An enticing, super-nutritious, gluten-free, protein-rich soup for monsoon and winter

Makes: 4 cups; Soaking time: 6–8 hours; Cooking time: 25 minutes; Effect on doshas: P-

Ingredients

- ¼ cup proso millet
- 2 tsp coconut oil
- ½ tsp dill seeds
- ½ cup carrots, peeled, chopped into ½-inch pieces
- ½ cup pumpkin, peeled, seeds removed, chopped into ½-inch pieces
- ½ cup fennel bulb, finely chopped
- 1 garlic clove, peeled, crushed
- 2½ cups water
- ½ tsp roasted cumin powder
- ½ tsp black pepper, coarsely ground
- ¼ tsp rock salt, or as per taste
- ½ cup coconut milk
- 2 tsp coriander, finely chopped

Method

- Wash and soak the proso millet in 1 cup water for 6–8 hours. Then discard the water.
- In a kadai, heat the coconut oil. When the oil becomes hot, add the dill seeds, millets, chopped carrots, pumpkin, fennel and garlic and sauté for 5–7 minutes.
- Then add water, cover and cook the vegetables on a moderate flame until tender. This should take about 15–20 minutes.
- Now add the cumin, black pepper, salt and coconut milk and continue to heat on a low flame for 1–2 minutes. Then remove from the heat. Let it cool down a bit, then blend it using a hand blender. Add coriander leaves and serve.

Note

- You can replace pumpkin with squash.

30. Amaranth Veggies

A yummy and healthy vegan superfood prepared with vegetables and mild spices, this is a satisfying and convenient lunch box recipe.

Makes: 1¼ cups; Soaking time: Overnight; Cooking time: 25–30 minutes; Effect on doshas: P-

Ingredients

- ½ cup amaranth
- 1 tsp fresh unsalted butter or ghee
- 2 tsp almonds and pecans, chopped
- 1 tsp raisins and seedless dates, finely chopped
- 1 tsp coriander seeds
- ½ tsp fennel seeds
- 1-inch cinnamon stick
- 1 tsp coconut oil
- ½ cup vegetables (a mix of any of these—squash, fennel or celery, carrot, asparagus, green beans), chopped into ½-inch pieces
- ¼ tsp rock salt, or as per taste
- 2 tsp coconut, grated (optional)
- 1 tsp mint leaves, finely chopped
- 3–4 saffron threads
- 2 green cardamoms
- ½ tsp turmeric powder
- 1 cup water
- 1 tsp parsley, finely chopped
- 1 tsp coriander, finely chopped

Method

- Wash and soak the amaranth in 2 cups of water overnight. Then discard the water.
- In a skillet or wok, add the butter or ghee and when it gets hot, roast the nuts and dry fruits and keep them aside. Now in the same skillet, add the coriander seeds, fennel seeds and cinnamon and sauté for a minute in the remaining butter/ghee. Then add the coconut oil, chopped vegetables and salt and sauté on a moderate flame for 7–10 minutes or until the vegetables are soft. Keep them aside.
- Take a pressure cooker or a thick-bottomed vessel, add the soaked amaranth, grated coconut, mint leaves, saffron, green cardamom and turmeric powder along with 1 cup of water and cook on a moderate flame for 3–4 whistles. If cooking in an open vessel, add an additional ¼ cup of water and cook for about 25 minutes until the amaranth is soft and well-cooked.
- Add the sautéed vegetables along with the spices to the cooked grain and mix well using a ladle. Sprinkle with parsley, coriander, roasted nuts and dry fruits and serve.

Note

- Pearl barley or quinoa or basmati rice can be used instead of amaranth. If you are using quinoa or basmati rice, wash and soak it in water for 30 minutes prior to cooking. However, if you are using pearl barley, wash it and soak it in water overnight.

31. Coco–Quinoa Rice

A satiating, gluten-free, high-fibre, high-protein recipe containing quinoa, coconut and spices

Makes: 1½ cups; Soaking time: 25 minutes; Preparation time: 30 minutes; Effect on doshas: P- V-

Ingredients

- ½ cup quinoa
- 1 cup water
- 1 tsp coconut oil
- ½ tsp mustard seeds
- 1-inch piece cinnamon stick
- 2 cloves
- 2 green cardamoms
- ½ cup coconut, grated
- ¼ tsp rock salt

Method

- Wash the quinoa in water and soak it for 30 minutes. Then discard the water.
- Add the quinoa to a saucepan along with 1 cup of water and cook for about 20 minutes on a low flame. Heat the oil in a skillet. Add the mustard seeds and when they splutter, add the cinnamon stick, cloves and cardamom and sauté for a minute.
- Then add the coconut and sauté for another minute.
- Add the salt and the cooked quinoa. Toss it and serve.

32. Carrot Yoghurt

A cooling recipe to be enjoyed in summertime, this carrot yoghurt is power packed with probiotics, protein and vitamins.

Makes: 2 cups; Preparation time: 15 minutes; Effect on doshas: P-

Ingredients

- 1 cup low-fat yoghurt
- ¼ cup carrot, peeled, grated

- ¼ cup cucumber, skin removed, finely chopped
- 6 tsp coriander, finely chopped
- ¼ tsp rock salt, or as per taste

Method

- In a bowl, add the yoghurt, whisk it and add the grated carrots, finely chopped cucumber, coriander and salt. Mix well and serve.

Note

- You can also use mung beans soaked overnight in water and pomegranate arils instead of carrots and cucumber in the recipe. If using soaked mung beans and pomegranate, this recipe will help balance the Kapha and Pitta doshas.

33. Purple Cabbage Stir-Fry

A mildly-spiced and sautéed cabbage recipe that is ready in 25 minutes

Makes: 2½ cups; Preparation time: 25 minutes; Effect on doshas: P-

Ingredients

- ¼ cup coconut, grated
- ¼ tsp cumin seeds
- 2 garlic pods, peeled, roughly chopped
- ¼ tsp turmeric powder
- 2 tsp coconut oil
- 3 cups purple cabbage, finely chopped
- ¼ cup shallots, finely chopped
- ¼ tsp rock salt, or as per taste

Method

- In a blender, add the coconut, cumin seeds, garlic pods and turmeric and pulse for 20–30 seconds.
- Heat the oil in a pan, then add the shallots and sauté them for 4–5 minutes, until they are soft and translucent. Then add the chopped cabbage and cover and cook on a moderate flame for 12–15 minutes.
- Then add the coconut mixture and sauté for a minute. Add the salt. Then cover with a lid and cook for 5–7 minutes while stirring occasionally. Serve with rice or flatbreads.

Note

- You can also use white cabbage/pumpkin/carrots/beans as your vegetable of choice.

34. Sautéed Brussels Sprouts

A crispy and caramelized recipe that is simple and quick to prepare

Makes: 2 cups; Preparation time: 30 minutes; Effect on doshas: P- K-

Ingredients

- 2 cups brussels sprouts
- ¼ tsp rock salt, or as per taste
- 2 tsp lemon juice
- 2 tsp water, if needed
- 2 tsp ghee
- 1 pinch asafoetida
- 1 bay leaf
- 1 tsp garlic, finely chopped
- 1 cup onion, finely chopped
- 1 tsp cumin powder
- ¼ tsp cinnamon powder

- 2 tsp coriander powder
- 1 tsp turmeric powder
- 1 tsp black pepper powder
- ½ tsp cardamom powder

Method

- Trim off the stems of the brussels sprouts. Wash them in water. Cut the sprouts lengthwise into two halves. Now slice them crosswise into thin pieces. Loosen the pieces.
- Transfer the brussels sprouts to a skillet. Add the salt and lemon juice. Mix well and cook on a low flame for 10 minutes, keeping the skillet covered with a lid. Stir occasionally to prevent them from sticking to the bottom of the skillet. If needed, you may add 2 tsp of water to cook the sprouts till they are soft. Then remove them from the heat.
- Heat another pan, add the ghee and when it becomes hot, add the asafoetida, bay leaf, garlic and onion and sauté for 4–5 minutes. Then add the cumin, cinnamon, coriander and turmeric powders and sauté for a minute more.
- Add the cooked brussels sprouts and cook for 2–3 minutes.
- Add the black pepper and cardamom powders and toss well. Serve with rice or flatbreads.

35. Steamed Carrots

A super easy recipe where spices are simply sprinkled on steamed carrots and served

Makes: 1 cup; Preparation time: 20 minutes; Effect on doshas: P- V-

Ingredients

- 1 cup carrots, peeled, cut into ¼-inch pieces
- 4 tsp water
- 1 tsp cumin powder

- ½ tsp coriander powder
- ¼ tsp fennel powder
- ¼ tsp black pepper powder
- ¼ tsp turmeric powder
- Rock salt as per taste
- 1 tsp coconut oil (optional)

Method

- Heat a skillet, add the carrots and sprinkle 4 tsp water. Cover with a lid and cook on a moderate flame for 7–10 minutes or until the carrots become soft. Make sure to stir in between to prevent the contents from sticking to the bottom of the skillet.
- Transfer the cooked carrots to a plate, sprinkle with cumin, coriander, turmeric, fennel and black pepper powders and salt. Serve with rice or flatbreads.
- If you want, you can pour 1 tsp of coconut oil over the steamed carrots after adding the spices and enjoy this dish fresh.

Note

- You can replace carrots with beans, cauliflower, broccoli, beets or peas.

36. Spinach Gravy

An aromatic recipe that is loaded with nutritious spinach simmered in a buttery coconut cream

Makes: 1 cup; Preparation time: 10 minutes; Effect on doshas: P-

Ingredients

- 6 tsp coconut, shredded (you can also use 4 tsp coconut milk instead)
- 6 tsp yoghurt
- 1 tsp cumin seeds (divided into ½ tsp + ½ tsp)
- 1 tsp coconut oil

- 1 cup spinach leaves, finely chopped
- 6 tsp capsicum, finely chopped
- ¼ tsp rock salt, or as per taste
- 2 tsp water

Method

- Add the shredded coconut, yoghurt and ½ tsp cumin seeds to the mixer and grind them.
- Heat coconut oil in a skillet, add ½ tsp cumin seeds and sauté for 20–30 seconds. Then add the spinach and capsicum and sauté for 3–4 minutes.
- Now add salt and 2 tsp water, cover and cook for another 3–4 minutes. Then add the ground coconut mixture and salt, mix well and simmer for 2 minutes. Remove from the heat and serve with rice or flatbreads or savoury pancakes.

Note

- You can also prepare the above recipe using beets, cucumbers, carrots or okra instead of spinach. If using beets or carrots, peel and grate them before you use them. If using cucumbers, peel and finely chop them before using. If using okra, wash and chop the okra into ½-inch pieces. But the okra should be cooked for a longer time, say 10–12 minutes.

37. Lentil–Amaranth Curry

A simple and flavourful high-protein recipe for sensitive tummies that can't handle spicy curries

Makes: 1½ cups; Soaking time: 30 minutes; Preparation time: 20 minutes; Effect on doshas: P-

Ingredients

- ¼ cup yellow mung

- 1¼ cups water (divided into 1 cup + ¼ cup)
- 1 cup amaranth leaves, finely chopped
- 1 tsp ghee
- 1 tsp cumin seeds, crushed
- 6 tsp shallots, finely chopped
- ½ tsp fresh ginger, grated
- 1 garlic clove, peeled, finely chopped
- ¼ tsp rock salt, or as per taste

Method

- Wash and soak the yellow mung in water for 30 minutes. Then discard the water.
- In a saucepan, cook the yellow mung with 1 cup of water until it is cooked to a soft consistency. This should take about 15 minutes.
- Heat ¼ cup of water in a saucepan and add the amaranth leaves. Cover and cook on low to medium heat for about 5–7 minutes.
- Heat ghee in a kadai and add cumin seeds and sauté for 30 seconds. Now add the shallots and sauté for 2 minutes. Then add the fresh ginger and garlic and sauté for a minute. Now add the cooked amaranth leaves and cooked mung along with the residual water. Let it come to a boil.
- Add the rock salt and mix well. Then remove from the heat and serve with rice or flatbreads.

Note

- You can use lettuce instead of amaranth leaves in this recipe.

38. Pumpkin Curry

A simple yet satisfying tangy curry packed with flavour

Makes: 1 cup; Preparation time: 30 minutes; Effect on doshas: P-

Ingredients

- ½ cup water
- 1 cup pumpkin, skin and seeds removed, chopped into 1-inch long pieces
- 1 tsp tamarind paste
- 1 tsp jaggery powder
- 1 tsp black lentil powder
- ½ tsp turmeric powder
- 2 tsp ghee
- 1 tsp cumin seeds
- ¼ tsp fenugreek seeds
- ¼ tsp rock salt, or as per taste

Method

- In a saucepan, add the water and pumpkin pieces. Cover and cook it on a low flame for about 20 minutes.
- Meanwhile, mix the tamarind paste, jaggery and black lentil flour in a bowl. Now add this to the pumpkin along with the turmeric powder. Cover with a lid and continue cooking for 5 minutes or until the water has evaporated. Then open the lid. If the water is not yet evaporated, then cook without the lid for 3–5 minutes.
- Heat the ghee in another pan, add the cumin and fenugreek seeds and sauté for 1–2 minutes. Mix in the salt. Add this to the cooked pumpkin, toss and serve.

Note

- You can use yoghurt instead of tamarind paste.

39. Mung–Ginger Pudding

A not-too-sweet, aromatic and delightful nutrient-dense dessert

Makes: 4 cups; Soaking time: 1 hour; Preparation time: 40 minutes; Effect on doshas: P- V- K+

Ingredients

- 1 cup yellow mung
- ½ cup almonds
- 1 cup milk
- ¾ cup cow's ghee
- ¼ cup dry ginger powder
- 1 cup rock sugar powder
- ¼ tsp nutmeg powder
- ¼ tsp cumin powder
- ¼ tsp black pepper powder
- ¼ tsp coriander powder
- ¼ tsp long pepper powder
- ¼ tsp cinnamon powder
- ¼ tsp cardamom powder
- ¼ tsp clove powder
- 6–8 tsp water

Method

- Wash and soak the mung in water for at least 1 hour. Then discard the water and grind the mung to a paste using a mixer-grinder with 6–8 tsp water.
- Grind the almonds to a powder using a mixer-grinder.
- Boil the milk and keep it aside.
- In a pan, heat the ghee and fry the mung paste for 20 minutes. When the mung is brownish, add the dry ginger powder, ground almonds and sugar. Mix well.
- Now add the milk little by little while stirring well. Keep cooking on a low flame until the mixture thickens and all the contents are well cooked.

- Add all the other spice powders, mix well, remove from the heat and serve hot.

40. Mishti Lush

A thick, creamy, cooling and delicious dessert

Makes: 2 cups; Setting time: 1–2 hours; Preparation time: 5 minutes; Chilling time: 1–2 hours; Effect on doshas: P- V- K+

Ingredients

- 1 cup pumpkin, peeled, seeds removed, roughly chopped
- 1½ cups cow's milk
- 1 cup full-fat fresh yoghurt (should not be sour)
- ¾ cup rock sugar powder
- ¼ tsp cardamom powder
- 2 pinches clove powder
- 2 pinches black pepper powder

Method

- Grind the pumpkin in a mixer-grinder to a smooth consistency. Then filter and squeeze it using a ladle to extract as much juice as possible.
- Now add the rock sugar powder to the pumpkin juice and heat in a kadai on a medium flame while stirring continuously until the sugar is fully dissolved.
- Continue cooking until the mixture thickens, that is, about 10–12 minutes. Then remove from the heat.
- In another kadai or thick-bottomed vessel, boil the milk on a moderate to low flame until the milk is reduced to half its quantity. Now remove from the heat and stir in the pumpkin syrup. Let it become lukewarm.
- Take the yoghurt in a bowl and whisk it. Now add this yoghurt to the milk-pumpkin syrup mixture. Also add the cardamom, clove and black pepper powders. Mix using a ladle just once.

Now pour this into small cups, preferably made of clay. Tie the mouth of the cups with a muslin cloth. Leave them out overnight. After that you can refrigerate the dish for a minimum of 1–2 hours before consumption. This has to be consumed within 1–2 days.

41. Pumpkin–Yoghurt Summer Treat

An extremely hydrating and thirst-quenching summer treat that is a great alternative to cold drinks

Makes: 2 cups; Preparation time: 5 minutes; Effect on doshas: P- K+

Ingredients
- 2 cups yellow pumpkin, skin and seeds removed, roughly chopped
- 1 cup fresh yoghurt (should not be sour)
- ¼ tsp cardamom powder
- ¼ tsp cinnamon powder
- 1 tsp palm sugar, or as per taste (you can also use rock sugar)

Method
- Add the pumpkin, yoghurt, cardamom and cinnamon powders and palm or rock sugar to a vessel and blend using a hand blender. Serve immediately.

Note
- The quantity of rock sugar can be adjusted based on the sweetness of the pumpkin.

42. Almond Treat

A nutty recipe that improves brain function

Makes: 2 cups; Soaking time: Overnight; Preparation time: 30 minutes; Effect on doshas: P- V- K+

Ingredients

- 1 cup almonds
- 6 tsp water
- 2 cups + 2 tsp milk
- 5–6 strands saffron
- 6 tsp ghee
- ¼ cup rock sugar powder
- 10–12 raisins, finely chopped
- 10–12 pistachios, finely chopped

Method

- Soak almonds in water overnight. The next morning, peel off the skin and grind the almonds with 6 tsp water to a smooth paste in a mixer-grinder.
- Soak the saffron in 2 tsp milk.
- Boil 2 cups of milk in a saucepan.
- Meanwhile, heat a skillet and add the ghee to it. When the ghee becomes hot, add the almond paste and fry for about 2–3 minutes. No need to brown the almonds.
- Slowly add the hot milk to this mixture while stirring constantly.
- Let the mixture come to a boil. Simmer and cook it until it thickens to a semi-solid consistency. This should take about 20–25 minutes. Keep stirring in between to prevent the contents from sticking to the bottom.
- Now add the sugar and let it cook for 2 more minutes. Add the saffron soaked in milk, chopped raisins and pistachios.
- If you prefer a semi-liquid consistency, you may add ½ a cup of warm milk at this stage. Mix well and consume.

43. Amaranth Delight

A deliciously flavourful gluten-free dessert

Makes: 2 cups; Preparation time: 30 minutes; Effect on doshas: P-

Ingredients
- 1 pinch saffron
- 2 tsp + 2 cups milk
- ½ cup amaranth seeds
- 1 tsp ghee
- 5–7 raisins
- ¼ tsp cardamom powder
- 5–6 almonds, chopped lengthwise
- 1 tsp rock sugar powder

Method
- Soak the saffron strands in 2 tsp milk and keep it aside.
- Heat a skillet and dry roast the amaranth seeds in it on a moderate flame for about 5–7 minutes. When they pop, remove them from the heat and transfer them to a plate. If you are using a small skillet you can also dry roast the amaranth seeds in 2–3 batches.
- Heat a pan, add 2 cups of milk to it and when it comes to a boil, add the amaranth seeds. Cook on a moderate flame until the amaranth seeds are well-cooked. This will take approximately 25 minutes. The amaranth should be soft, sticky and of a gelatinous consistency when squeezed between your fingers.
- Now add the raisins to the cooked amaranth. Also add the saffron soaked in milk, cardamom powder, almonds and rock sugar powder. Mix well and serve.

44. Lapsika

A super healthy and sweet snack that is perfect for growing children

Makes: ½ cup; Preparation time: 25–30 minutes; Effect on doshas: P- V- K+

Ingredients

- ¼ cup milk
- ½ cup rock sugar powder
- ½ cup ghee
- ½ cup wholewheat flour
- 2–3 pinches cardamom powder
- 2 pinches black pepper powder

Method

- Heat milk in a saucepan and add rock sugar powder to it. Mix well and keep aside.
- In a thick-bottomed vessel, fry the wholewheat flour in ghee on low heat until the flour changes to a deep brown colour and becomes aromatic. This should take about 15–20 minutes.
- Slowly add the hot milk mixed with the rock sugar powder to the wheat, while stirring to prevent lumps. Keep cooking on a low flame till the mixture reaches a thick but soft, moist consistency, like that of a pudding. After the mixture absorbs all the milk, there will be a change in texture too. This will take about 3–5 minutes.
- Then add the cardamom and black pepper powders. Mix well and serve while it is warm.
- The mixture will solidify and thicken when left for a long time. If you want to soften the consistency, you may add some hot water or hot milk and stir well to soften it before serving.

Notes

- Do not use cold milk as it might cause lumps.
- If you are lactose intolerant, use coconut milk or hot water instead of hot milk.

45. Coco Ksheera

Treat yourself to this nourishing nectar

Makes: ½ cup; Preparation time: 25 minutes; Effect on doshas: P- V-

Ingredients

- 1 tsp ghee
- ¼ cup coconut, grated/scraped
- ¾ cup milk
- 6 tsp rock sugar powder

Method

- Heat the ghee in a thick-bottomed vessel. Add the coconut and fry for 3–4 minutes on low heat. Do not brown the coconut.
- Now add the milk and sugar and cook on a low flame for about 15–20 minutes until the coconut is completely cooked and the mixture thickens. Keep stirring occasionally.

Note

- This recipe can be prepared with ash gourd pieces instead of grated coconut.

46. Avocado Bites

A cool, refreshing and easy-to-make avocado dessert

Makes: 4; Preparation time: 20 minutes; Drying time: 1–2 days; Effect on doshas: V- P- K+

Ingredients

- 2 ripe avocados
- ½ tsp ghee + more for greasing
- ¼ cup rock sugar
- 2 pinches cardamom powder

Method

- Remove the skin and seeds of the avocados. Then scoop out the flesh using a spoon and grind it in a blender to make a paste. Do not add any water.
- Grease a flat plate with ghee and keep it aside.
- Heat a skillet, add the avocado pulp and the sugar. Keep the skillet on a low flame for 15 minutes, stirring once in a while. Bubbles will start forming and the mixture will thicken.
- At this stage, add the cardamom powder and mix well.
- Transfer the avocado paste to the greased plate and spread it uniformly. The thickness should be about 1 inch.
- When it cools down to room temperature, cover the plate with a cheesecloth and sun-dry it for 1–2 days, or you may keep it inside the house until it dries, which might take about 2–3 days.
- When completely dried, cut it into squares. Store it in a moisture-free airtight container at room temperature for up to 7 days.

47. Coco–Butter Bars

A soft, chewy and buttery dessert for coconut lovers

Makes: 4; Cooking time: 20 minutes; Setting time: 5–7 minutes; Effect on doshas: P- V-

Ingredients

- ½ cup coconut, shredded
- ½ cup rock sugar powder
- 1 cup milk
- 7 tsp ghee (divided into 6 tsp + 1 tsp)
- ¼ tsp cardamom powder
- 10 pistachios, coarsely chopped

Method

- Combine the coconut, rock sugar, milk and 6 tsp ghee in a thick-bottomed vessel and cook on a low flame for about 15–20 minutes until the mixture attains a semi-solid consistency while stirring periodically to prevent the contents from sticking to the bottom.
- Now add the cardamom powder and mix well.
- Grease a plate with 1 tsp ghee and transfer the prepared mixture on to it. Set well, using a ladle to smooth it into a block with about 1 inch height.
- Sprinkle the chopped pistachios on the top layer of the block and press down gently using a ladle. Allow it to set for about 5–7 minutes.
- When the block is still lukewarm, cut it into square-shaped pieces using a knife.
- When it cools down to room temperature, transfer it to a moisture-free airtight container. This can be stored in the refrigerator for up to 3 days.

48. Beet Bars

This beet bar fights fatigue and restores your energy levels.

Makes: 6; Cooking time: 20 minutes; Setting time: 7–10 minutes; Effect on doshas: P- V-

Ingredients

- 3 tsp ghee (divided into 2 tsp +1 tsp)
- 1 cup beetroot, grated
- 1 cup coconut, grated
- 1½ cups sugar
- ¼ tsp cardamom powder

Method

- Heat 2 tsp ghee in a pan, then add the grated beets and coconut. Sauté on a moderate flame for about 10–12 minutes or until the raw smell is gone.
- Now add the sugar and cardamom powder and mix well. Cook on a low flame for 3–5 minutes. Keep stirring continuously.
- Grease a plate with 1 tsp ghee. Transfer the beetroot mix on to the plate and spread it evenly, making a layer that is approximately 1 inch in thickness.
- When it cools down to lukewarm temperature, cut it into square pieces. You can store it in an airtight container at room temperature for about 7 days and in the refrigerator for up to 15 days.

49. Dessert Balls

This sweet snack is energizing and nutritious.

Makes: 10; Preparation time: 40 minutes; Effect on doshas: P- V- K+

Ingredients

- ¼ cup black lentil powder
- ¼ cup wheat flour
- ¼ cup barley flour
- ¼ cup rice powder
- ¼ cup black pepper powder

- ¾ cup cow's ghee + more for greasing
- 1¼ cups rock sugar powder
- 6¼ cups water

Method

- Mix the black lentil, wheat flour, barley, rice and black pepper powders in a bowl.
- Heat the ghee in a kadai and add the powders. Fry on mild to moderate heat for about 12–15 minutes or until the powders emit a good aroma.
- Heat the water in a saucepan or a kettle and add it to the kadai in parts. Cook on a low flame and keep stirring in between to prevent chunks from forming. Cook until the mixture attains a semi-solid dough-like mass. This should take about 12–15 minutes.
- Then add the rock sugar powder and stir for about 2–3 minutes.
- Transfer it to a bowl and when the mixture is lukewarm, make golf-sized balls of dough.
- If you think the mixture is dry or is sticking to your hands, you can grease your hands with a little ghee.
- Once the balls are made and they cool down to room temperature, they can be stored in a moisture-free airtight container at room temperature for 5 days or in the refrigerator for up to 10 days. Consume one ball a day.

Note

- You can also consume this like a pudding instead of making balls.

50. Millet Sweet Balls

An immunity-boosting, gluten-free, protein- and fibre-rich sweet that can be prepared quickly

Makes: 5; Preparation time: 20 minutes; Effect on doshas: P-

Ingredients
- ½ cup jaggery powder
- ½ cup water
- 1 cup foxtail millet flour
- 6 tsp ghee + more for greasing
- 10–12 raisins
- 2 pinches cardamom powder

Method
- Heat the jaggery powder with the water in a pan and let it come to a boil. Then strain it using a cloth strainer. Keep the strained syrup aside.
- Dry roast the foxtail millet flour on medium heat in a hot pan for 5–7 minutes while stirring in between.
- Then add the jaggery syrup and mix well so that no lumps form in the batter.
- Meanwhile, heat the ghee in a skillet and add the raisins to it. Sauté for 2 minutes or until the raisins are plump.
- Add this to the flour mixture along with cardamom powder and heat for 3–5 minutes or until the mixture solidifies and does not stick to the pan.
- When the mixture becomes lukewarm, grease your hands with ghee. Take 6 tsp of this mixture and apply pressure evenly to make round balls. Repeat with the remaining flour mixture.
- This can be stored in an airtight moisture-free container for up to 10 days in the refrigerator.

RECIPES FOR KAPHA

1. Warming Ginger Infusion
2. Spicy Sweet Tea
3. Kokum Juice
4. Tangy Goji Drink
5. Green Energizer Juice
6. Wellness Shot
7. Jujube Juice
8. Warming Spring Beverage
9. Garlic Milk
10. Savoury Buttermilk
11. Horse Gram Porridge
12. Garlic Pesto
13. Tomato Pesto
14. Ridge Gourd Chutney
15. Mint–Tomato Dip
16. Strawberry Dip
17. Jaggery Spread
18. Tangy Ginger Relish
19. Sesame Spread
20. Sprouted Alfalfa Spread
21. Mashed Eggplant
22. Barley Buttermilk

23. Maize Porridge
24. Rye Porridge
25. Buckwheat Pancakes
26. Buckwheat Dumplings
27. Steamed Millet Flour
28. Mixed Veg Barley Flatbread
29. Spinach Flatbread
30. Maize Flatbread
31. Barley–Millet Fried Bread
32. Mung Salad
33. Millet–Rice Cake
34. Bean Salad
35. Fenugreek Chaat
36. Broccoli–Peas Soup
37. Protein Leek Soup
38. Amaranth Veggie Mix
39. Buckwheat Veggie Crunch
40. Millet Kitchari
41. Seasoned Yoghurt
42. Spinach Yoghurt
43. Yam Smash
44. Veg Stir-Fry
45. Eggplant Shallow Fry
46. Crunchy Amaranth Stir-Fry
47. Tangy Turnip
48. Peppery Curry
49. Healthy Modak
50. Millet Bars

1. Warming Ginger Infusion

This infusion helps to burn fat, regulate blood sugar, lower cholesterol, decrease arterial plaque, flush out toxins from the body and reduce water retention

Makes: 1 cup; Preparation time: 10 minutes; Effect on doshas: K- V- P+

Ingredients

- ¼-inch piece fresh ginger
- 2–3 lemongrass stalks
- ½-inch piece cinnamon
- 1 cup water

Method

- Wash and thinly slice the ginger.
- Wash and gently crush or press the lemongrass stalks using either your hands or the back of a knife.
- Crush the cinnamon stick using a hand pounder.
- Boil the water in a pan. Then add the ginger and cinnamon and cover with a lid. Let the spices steep for 5–7 minutes.
- Now place a cloth filter over a cup and filter the infusion. Drink it warm.

Note

- You may add 1 tsp honey when the infusion is warm if you wish for it to be sweet.

2. Spicy Sweet Tea

This tea helps clear nasal congestion, soothes the throat and aids in digestion

Makes: 1 cup; Preparation time: 10 minutes; Effect on doshas: K- P-

Ingredients

- 1 tsp black peppercorns
- 1-inch liquorice stick
- 1 cup water

Method

- Coarse grind the black pepper and liquorice using a hand pounder.
- Heat the water in a saucepan. When it comes to a boil, remove from the heat and add the black pepper and liquorice.
- Cover with a lid and leave it for 5–7 minutes. Then filter using a cloth filter and drink lukewarm.

Note

- Other spices/herbs that can be used to make an infusion are mentioned in the table below. Use one or more of these in combination.

Spices	Herbs
Fenugreek, Cloves, Cinnamon, Turmeric, Ginger	Triphala (Fruits of Haritaki, Bibhitaki and Amalaki), Punarnava (*Boerrhavia diffusa*), Shigru (*Moringa oleifera*)

3. Kokum Juice

A perfect drink for hot summer days when you want to refresh your body and mood

Makes: 2 cups; Soaking time: 4–5 hours (for dry kokum fruits) and 2 hours (for fresh kokum fruits); Preparation time: 20 minutes; Effect on doshas: K- P-

Ingredients

- 1 cup kokum fruits (fresh or dry)
- 2 cups water
- 1 cup rock sugar powder
- ¼ tsp cardamom powder
- 1 tsp roasted cumin seed powder
- Rock salt as per taste

Method

- Wash and soak the kokum fruits in water. You may also soak the dry fruits in water for 4–5 hours and then leave them in the fridge overnight and prepare the juice the next morning.
- Then rub the kokum fruits with your hands so that all the pulp comes out.
- Now filter the pulp using a cloth filter and add the other ingredients to the strained liquid. Mix well and serve.

Notes

- If you want, you may add more water to dilute the juice.
- You can also adjust the quantity of sugar based on your preference.

4. Tangy Goji Drink

A super-nutritious, sweet yet tangy, appetizing digestive drink

Makes: 2 cups; Soaking time: 5–6 hours; Preparation time: 10 minutes; Effect on doshas: K-

Ingredients

- ¼ cup goji berries
- ¼ cup seedless dates

- ¼ cup pomegranate arils
- ¼ cup raisins
- ¼ cup garcinia fruit
- 2 cups water
- 6 tsp rock sugar (optional)

Method

- Wash the goji berries, dates, raisins and garcinia fruit, and then add the pomegranate arils to it. Crush them using a hand pounder or blender. Transfer to a large bowl.
- Add water and leave it for 5–6 hours or overnight. If leaving overnight, place it in the refrigerator or store it in a clay pot at room temperature.
- Then churn the mixture using a hand churner or blender.
- Filter using a cloth filter, add the sugar, mix well and serve.

Note

- You can replace garcinia with tamarind fruits.

5. Green Energizer Juice

A power-packed veggie juice ideal for the morning hours or after exercise

Makes: 1 cup; Preparation time: 10 minutes; Effect on doshas: K-

Ingredients

- 1 stalk celery
- ½-inch piece ginger
- 1 bunch spinach/kale
- ¼ cup low-fat yoghurt
- ¼ cup water

Method

- Wash and roughly chop the celery.
- Wash and roughly chop the ginger and spinach (including stem)/kale (including stalk).
- Add the chopped celery, ginger, spinach/kale to a blender along with the low-fat yoghurt and grind it to a smooth consistency.
- Add water, mix well and consume.

Note

- You can use water instead of yoghurt.

6. Wellness Shot

A refreshing juice that boosts immunity and promotes healthy digestion

Makes: 2 cups; Soaking time: 10 minutes; Preparation time: 5 minutes; Effect on doshas: K-

Ingredients

- A handful of wheatgrass
- 1 apple, seed removed, roughly chopped
- ½-inch piece ginger, roughly chopped
- 1 cup water

Method

- Wash and soak the wheatgrass in a bowl of water for 10 minutes. Then drain and roughly chop the wheatgrass.
- In a blender, add the chopped apple, ginger, wheatgrass and 1 glass of water and grind for 2–3 minutes.
- Then squeeze the juice through a steel-mesh strainer and consume.

Note

- This should be consumed immediately after preparation otherwise it will turn bitter.

7. Jujube Juice

A delicious and nutritious drink that helps boost metabolism

Makes: 2 cups; Preparation time: 15 minutes; Effect on doshas: P- K-

Ingredients

- 1 cup ripe fruits of jujube
- 2 cups water (divided into 1 cup + 1 cup)
- 1 tsp rock sugar powder
- 2 pinches cinnamon powder
- 2 pinches cardamom powder
- 1 pinch bay leaf powder

Method

- Wash the jujube fruits and cook them in 1 cup of water over a low flame. When the fruits become soft (this will take about 10–12 minutes), remove them from the heat.
- Crush the fruits and filter them through a strainer.
- Add 1 cup of water to the strained liquid along with the rock sugar and the cinnamon, cardamom and bay leaf powders. Serve.

Notes

- You can use cranberries instead of jujube fruits.
- If you are using dry jujube fruits or cranberries, you have to soak them in 1 cup of hot water for about 2–3 hours before you cook them. Then follow the procedure mentioned in the recipe.

8. Warming Spring Beverage

A healthy, warm and comforting spiced milk, this beverage is best consumed in spring to fight against allergies.

Makes: 1 cup; Preparation time: 15 minutes; Effect on doshas: K- V-

Ingredients

- 3–4 black peppercorns
- ½-inch piece cinnamon stick
- 2 cloves
- 1 cup goat's milk or skimmed milk
- ¼ tsp turmeric paste or powder

Method

- Crush the black peppercorns, cinnamon stick and cloves using a hand pounder.
- Bring the milk to a boil in a pan. Add the other ingredients and stir well for a minute. Remove from the heat. Filter and consume.

Note

- If you wish, you may add 1 tsp honey after preparing the drink, when the milk is lukewarm.

9. Garlic Milk

A flavourful medicinal drink for relief from aches and pains, and for improved joint and heart health

Makes: 1 cup; Preparation time: 10 minutes; Effect on doshas: K- V-

Ingredients

- 5 garlic cloves, skin peeled

- 1 cup milk
- 1 cup water

Method

- Wash and crush the garlic using a hand pounder.
- In a saucepan, add the milk, water and crushed garlic. Heat it over a low flame until it reduces to half the quantity, that is, 1 cup.
- Filter and enjoy the drink when it is lukewarm.

Note

- If you wish, you can add 1 tsp jaggery powder for a touch of sweetness.

10. Savoury Buttermilk

An appetizing and digestive recipe to help relieve colicky pain and flatulence

Makes: 1 cup; Preparation time: 5 minutes; Effect on doshas: V- K-

Ingredients

- 1 cup low-fat buttermilk
- ¼ tsp dry ginger powder
- Rock salt as per taste

Method

- Pour the buttermilk into a cup, add the other ingredients, mix well and serve.

Note

- If the recipe is prepared with 2 pinches of asafoetida and ½ tsp of cumin powder instead of ginger powder, it will help improve digestion and relieve haemorrhoids and dysentery.

11. Horse Gram Porridge

Often on the path of weight loss, there is a desire to eat something sweet—this is the perfect recipe to satiate that craving.

Makes: 20 servings; Preparation time: 30–35 minutes; Effect on doshas: K-

Ingredients

- ¼ cup wholegrain barley
- ¼ cup horse gram
- 2 tsp flaxseeds
- 2 tsp cumin seeds
- 2 tsp black pepper
- 2 tsp dry ginger powder
- ¼ cup jaggery powder

Method

- Heat a pan and dry roast the barley over low heat until it turns light brown in colour and releases a nutty aroma, that is, for about 7–10 minutes. Now transfer it to a plate.
- In the same pan, dry roast the horse gram till golden brown and transfer it to the same plate as the barley.
- Next, dry roast the flaxseeds, cumin seeds and black pepper together for 3–5 minutes, until they release an aroma, and transfer them to the same plate.
- Allow all the ingredients to cool down to room temperature. Then grind them together using a mixer-grinder to make a fine powder.
- Now add the dry ginger and jaggery powders and mix well.
- Transfer the mixture into an airtight container and store in a cool and dry place. If prepared well and stored without any moisture, this stays good for up to 3 months.

- To make the drink, heat 1 cup of water in a saucepan and add 2 tsp of this mix and cook it over moderate heat. The mixture will come to a boil. Continue cooking for 5 more minutes while stirring occasionally. Remove from the heat and consume when it is lukewarm.

Note

- You can replace horse gram with kidney beans in this recipe.

12. Garlic Pesto

A spicy and tasty pesto that is also good for aches and pains

Makes: ½ cup; Preparation time: 5 minutes; Effect on doshas: K- V-

Ingredients

- 12 medium-sized garlic cloves, skin peeled, roughly chopped
- 4 tsp jaggery powder
- 4 tsp sesame oil

Method

- Add the garlic to a blender along with the jaggery powder and the sesame oil and grind to a smooth paste.
- This recipe complements many vegetarian and non-vegetarian foods that are heavy to digest.

Note

- This recipe is not suitable for those suffering from acid reflux.

13. Tomato Pesto

This pesto is incredibly beneficial for your health as it protects your body cells from damage.

Makes: ¾ cup; Preparation time: 10 minutes; Effect on doshas: K- V-

Ingredients

- 4 tsp seedless dates, finely chopped
- 1½ tsp sesame oil
- ¼ tsp mustard seeds
- 3–4 curry leaves
- 1 cup tomatoes, skin peeled, finely chopped
- ¼ tsp rock salt, or as per taste
- ¼ tsp cumin powder
- ¼ tsp coriander powder
- ¼ tsp fennel seed powder
- ¼ tsp fenugreek powder

Method

- Crush the dates using a hand pounder to make a paste. Alternatively, you can also use a mixer-grinder.
- Heat a frying pan and add oil. When the oil is hot, add the mustard seeds. When it pops, add the curry leaves, tomatoes and salt. Cover and cook for 5 to 7 minutes while stirring once every minute. The tomatoes should become soft and well cooked. Then add the spice powders (cumin, coriander, fennel, fenugreek) and date paste. Mix well and continue to cook for 2 more minutes but without the lid.
- Serve with dumplings, savoury cakes or pancakes.

Notes

- You can use sweet beets instead of tomatoes. You can either grate the beets or finely chop them before using. However, if you use chopped beets, after cooking, you need to let the beets cool down to room temperature and then grind to a paste in a mixer-grinder.
- If you're using sweet beets, you do not have to use dates in the recipe.

- Also, when beets are used, the recipe will be beneficial for balancing Pitta and Vata doshas.

14. Ridge Gourd Chutney

Although this spread is an acquired taste, it is good for you as it is low in calories and boosts metabolism.

Makes: 1 cup; Preparation time: 20 minutes; Effect on doshas: K-

Ingredients

- 1¼ cups ridge gourd, outer skin scraped, roughly cut into pieces
- ¼ cup capsicum, seeds removed, roughly chopped
- 3 tsp roasted Bengal gram
- 3 garlic cloves, peeled, roughly chopped
- 2 tsp water
- 1 tsp oil
- ½ tsp mustard seeds
- ½ tsp cumin seeds
- 5–6 curry leaves
- ½ tsp rock salt, or as per taste
- 1 tsp lemon juice

Method

- Grind the chopped ridge gourd, capsicum, Bengal gram and garlic together with 2 tsp water in a mixer-grinder.
- Heat the oil in a skillet and once it is hot, add the mustard seeds.
- When they splutter, add the cumin seeds and curry leaves, and when they are roasted, add the ground mixture, cover and cook on a medium flame for 5–7 minutes.
- Remove from the heat and add the salt and lemon juice. Mix well and use for dressing salads or serve with cooked quinoa or rice.

Note

- This can be stored in an airtight container in the refrigerator for 2–3 days.

15. Mint–Tomato Dip

A tangy and refreshing dip made with basic ingredients

Makes: ¾ cup; Preparation time: 5 minutes; Effect on doshas: V- K-

Ingredients

- ½ cup tomatoes, roughly chopped
- 6 tsp capsicum, finely chopped
- 2–3 black peppercorns
- 1 cup coriander leaves, roughly chopped
- 1 cup mint leaves, roughly chopped
- ¼ tsp rock salt, or as per taste

Method

- Grind all the ingredients together in a mixer-grinder to a fine paste and serve as a veggie dip.

Note

- This can be refrigerated for 2–3 days in an airtight container.

16. Strawberry Dip

This all-natural, home-made, finger-licking, low-sugar healthy dip is loaded with Vitamin C and powerful antioxidants and is quite easy to prepare.

Makes: 1 cup; Preparation time: 15 minutes; Effect on doshas: V- K-

Ingredients

- 1 cup strawberries, roughly chopped
- 1 tsp ginger, grated
- ½ tsp fresh turmeric, grated
- 2 tsp water
- ¼ cup jaggery powder
- ¼ tsp black pepper powder
- ½ tsp cumin powder
- 3–4 pinches salt, or as per taste
- ¼ tsp coconut oil
- 1 tsp lemon juice

Method

- Heat a saucepan and add the strawberries, ginger, turmeric, water and jaggery to it. Cook on a moderate flame until the strawberries have softened and the jaggery has melted. This should take about 5–7 minutes.
- Now add the black pepper powder, cumin powder and rock salt and keep stirring the mixture for 2–3 minutes.
- Then remove from the heat, pour in the coconut oil and lemon juice, mix well and serve.
- This can be used as a dip or spread over any kind of flatbreads or pancakes.

17. Jaggery Spread

A multivitamin booster that has a unique and unbeatable taste

Makes: ½ cup; Preparation time: 5 minutes; Effect on doshas: V- K-

Ingredients

- ¼ cup ghee
- ¼ cup jaggery powder
- ½ tsp dry ginger powder
- ½ tsp black pepper powder
- ½ tsp bishop's weed powder

Method

- Heat the ghee in a pan, add the other ingredients to it and when the mixture becomes pasty, remove it from the heat. This should take approximately 3–5 minutes.
- Now mix well to get a fine paste. You can enjoy it as a spread on pancakes or flatbreads.

18. Tangy Ginger Relish

A finger-licking, delicious appetizer with the sourness of tamarind, the sweetness of natural sugar and the spiciness of ginger

Makes: ½ cup; Preparation time: 25 minutes; Effect on doshas: V- K-

Ingredients

- 2 tsp sesame oil
- 1 tsp mustard seeds
- 5–6 curry leaves
- 6 tsp fresh ginger, grated
- 1 green chilli, finely chopped
- ¼ cup tamarind paste
- ¼ cup water
- ¼ cup jaggery powder

- ¼ tsp rock salt, or as per taste
- ¼ tsp fenugreek seed powder
- ¼ tsp black pepper powder

Method

- Heat 2 tsp sesame oil in a pan and when it becomes hot, add the mustard seeds.
- When they splutter, add the curry leaves, grated ginger and finely chopped green chilli and sauté for a minute.
- Add the tamarind paste, water, jaggery and salt and boil over a medium flame for 15–20 minutes while stirring occasionally.
- When the mixture thickens and the oil starts to separate, remove from the heat.
- Add the fenugreek and black pepper powders and mix well.
- Serve with rice or flatbreads or pancakes.

Note

- This can be transferred to an airtight container when it cools down to room temperature and stored in the refrigerator for up to 15 days.

19. Sesame Spread

A perfect condiment to keep you warm in the winter

Makes: ½ cup; Preparation time: 5 minutes; Effect on doshas: V- K-

Ingredients

- ¼ cup sesame seeds
- 5 tsp lemon juice
- 1 tsp rock salt powder
- 5 tsp fresh ginger, grated

Method

- Grind the sesame seeds into a fine powder using a mixer-grinder or a hand pounder.
- Add the lemon juice, rock salt and grated ginger.
- Mix well and serve with pancakes or flatbreads. It can also be used as a dip when mixed with yoghurt or as a salad dressing.

Note

- If you feel the spread is too dry, you can add 1–2 tsp water.

20. Sprouted Alfalfa Spread

A quick-to-prepare and nutritious recipe with alfalfa sprouts, herbs and spices

Makes: 1 cup; Soaking time: Overnight; Preparation time: 5 minutes; Effect on doshas: K-

Ingredients

- 1 tsp fenugreek seeds
- 1 cup alfalfa sprouts (for details about how to make sprouts, see Pgs. 63–65)
- 1 tsp cumin seeds
- 1 tsp mustard seeds
- 1 tsp black peppercorns
- 5–6 fresh basil leaves
- 2 tsp water, or as needed
- 2 tsp lemon juice
- 1 tsp olive oil

Method

- Soak the fenugreek seeds in water overnight. The next morning, discard the water.
- In a bowl, mix the alfalfa sprouts, cumin seeds, mustard seeds, black peppercorns, fenugreek seeds and basil leaves. Now grind them to a smooth paste using a hand blender. You may add 2 tsp water to grind the mixture. Transfer to a bowl, add the lemon juice and olive oil, mix well and serve with rice or flatbreads.

Notes

- If you prefer a spicy flavour, you may add 1 dry red chilli instead of the black peppercorns.
- You can use clover sprouts or mung sprouts instead of alfalfa sprouts. You can also soak yellow mung in water overnight and use that instead.

21. Mashed Eggplant

A simple and delicious high-protein spread

Makes: 1 cup; Soaking time: Overnight; Preparation time: 20 minutes; Effect on doshas: K-

Ingredients

- ¼ cup chickpeas
- 1 small eggplant
- 2 cups water
- 6 tsp white sesame seeds
- 2 garlic cloves, peeled
- 2 tsp lemon juice
- 6 tsp sesame oil
- ¼ tsp rock salt
- 1 tsp parsley or basil, finely chopped

Method

- Wash and soak the chickpeas in water overnight. Then discard the water the next morning.
- Cook the chickpeas with 2 cups of water in a pressure cooker for 5–6 whistles.
- When the pressure goes off, remove the lid and strain the chickpeas.
- Rinse the eggplant under running water and dry it with a towel or paper napkin. Then turn on a burner to a medium flame and place the eggplant directly on the flame using tongs. After 2–3 minutes, use the tongs to turn the eggplant so that it is properly cooked. When the skin of the eggplant is fully burnt and flaky and the flesh is soft, remove it from the fire and place it on a plate. Let it cool down. This may take about 10 minutes. Then place the eggplant in a colander and rinse it gently while removing the skin.
- In a mixer-grinder, add the chickpeas, roasted eggplant, white sesame seeds, garlic, lemon juice, sesame oil and rock salt and grind into a fine paste.
- Garnish with parsley and serve with rice, quinoa, flatbreads or savoury pancakes. You can store this in the fridge for 2–3 days.

22. Barley Buttermilk

A super easy recipe with simple ingredients for a healthy boost of proteins, vitamins and minerals

Makes: 1 cup; Cooking time: 2–3 minutes; Resting time: 30 minutes; Preparation time: 10 minutes; Effect on doshas: K-

Ingredients

- 2 tsp barley flour
- 1 cup water
- 4 tsp yoghurt
- 2 shallots, finely chopped

- ½ tsp fresh ginger, grated
- ½ tsp roasted cumin seeds
- 1 tsp mint leaves, finely chopped
- 1 tsp carrot greens or basil leaves, finely chopped
- Salt as per taste (optional)

Method

- Heat a pan and dry roast the barley flour for 2–3 minutes. Then transfer it to a bowl.
- Heat the water in a pan and add it to the roasted barley flour. Mix well to prevent any lumps from forming. Cover with a lid and let it rest for 30 minutes.
- Then add all the other ingredients and blend using a hand blender. Serve.

23. Maize Porridge

One of the easiest and tastiest recipes in the book, this soft and creamy porridge boosts satiety, improves gut health and regulates energy balance.

Makes: 2 cups; Cooking time: 12 minutes; Resting time: 3–4 hours + overnight in the refrigerator; Preparation time: 10 minutes; Effect on doshas: K-

Ingredients

- ¼ cup maize flour
- 2 cups buttermilk (divided into 1 cup + 1 cup)
- 1 tsp sesame oil
- 1 pinch asafoetida
- ½ tsp cumin seeds
- ¼ tsp rock salt, or as per taste
- 1 tsp coriander leaves, finely chopped

Method

- In a bowl, add the maize flour. Then add 1 cup of buttermilk to it and mix well using a spatula or hand blender. There should be no lumps.
- Now transfer the mixture to a saucepan and cook it on a high flame while stirring constantly. When the mixture boils, reduce the flame and cook on a medium to low flame until the mixture thickens. This should take about 10–12 minutes. Stir occasionally to prevent lumps.
- Once the mixture attains a thick but flowing consistency, remove it from the heat.
- After cooking the maize porridge, you can also cover it with a lid and leave it at room temperature for about 3–4 hours and then refrigerate it overnight. The next day, the mixture would have thickened. Leave it outside at room temperature for about 30 minutes. Then add 1 more cup of buttermilk and blend using a hand blender.
- Heat the oil in a skillet and add the asafoetida and cumin seeds. Sauté for a minute and pour it into the mixture.
- Add salt and mix well. Garnish with coriander leaves and serve.

24. Rye Porridge

A nourishing and fulfilling breakfast recipe

Makes: 3 cups; Soaking time: Overnight; Cooking time: 25 minutes; Effect on doshas: K-

Ingredients

- ¼ cup rye
- ¼ cup black lentils (with skin)
- ½ tsp fenugreek seeds
- 3 garlic cloves, crushed
- 1½ cups water
- ¼ cup yoghurt
- ¼ tsp rock salt

Method

- Wash and soak the rye and black lentils separately in 1 cup of water each overnight. Then discard the water.
- Add the rye, black lentils, fenugreek, crushed garlic and water to a pressure cooker and cook for 5–6 whistles.
- When the pressure goes off, remove the lid.
- Whisk the yoghurt in a bowl and add it to the cooked millets.
- Add the salt, mix well and serve.

Note

- In this recipe, the rye can be replaced with barnyard millet.

25. Buckwheat Pancakes

A prebiotic, high-fibre recipe that is an ideal choice for weight loss

Makes: 4; Preparation time: 10 minutes; Resting time: 30 minutes; Cooking time: 25 minutes; Effect on doshas: K-

Ingredients

- ½ cup buckwheat flour
- ¼ cup chickpea flour
- 1 tsp semolina
- 6 tsp yoghurt
- 1¼ cups water
- ½ tsp fenugreek powder
- 2 pinches asafoetida
- 2 tsp capsicum, finely chopped
- ¼ tsp rock salt, or as per taste
- 6 tsp mustard/sesame oil

Method

- In a vessel, add the buckwheat flour, chickpea flour, semolina, yoghurt and water, then mix well using a ladle to make a smooth paste. Then add the fenugreek powder, asafoetida, capsicum and salt to it and mix well. There should be no lumps. Cover with a lid and keep it aside for 30 minutes.
- The batter should have a flowing consistency. If it is too thick, add a little water to adjust the consistency.
- Heat a tawa and grease it with oil. Pour a ladle full of batter into the tawa. Spread it into a circle to make a moderately thick disc and drizzle 1 tsp oil on the sides and the centre. Cover with a lid. After about 2–3 minutes, or when the upper surface of the pancake becomes partially cooked, flip and cook it on the other side for 3 minutes. Remove gently from the tawa and serve with pesto.

Note

- You can also use little millet flour instead of buckwheat flour. However, when you use little millet flour, add 3 tbsp rice flour to the recipe.

26. Buckwheat Dumplings

These dumplings are soft and delicious nutty little bites that serve as a filling comfort food.

Makes: 12; Preparation time: 15 minutes; Resting time: 15 minutes; Cooking time: 15 minutes; Effect on doshas: K-

Ingredients

- ½ cup buckwheat flour
- ¼ tsp rock salt, or as per taste
- 2 tsp sesame oil (divided into 1 tsp + 1 tsp)
- 1¼ cups water

- 2 pinches asafoetida
- ½ tsp mustard seeds
- 2 tsp coconut, grated

Method

- Mix the buckwheat flour and wheat flour in a bowl. Now dry roast the mix in a thick-bottomed vessel on a low flame for about 10–12 minutes until it emits a strong aroma. Then transfer it to a bowl. Add the salt and 1 tsp of sesame oil to it. Boil the water in a saucepan. Now add it little by little to the flour mix and knead well to make a dough. Cover with a lid and leave it for 10–15 minutes at room temperature. Then make small balls out of the dough (half the size of a lemon).
- Steam cook the balls in a steamer for 10–15 minutes. If your steamer capacity is limited, steam them in 2–3 batches.
- When all the balls are steamed, heat 1 tsp sesame oil in a pan, then add the asafoetida and the mustard seeds. When the mustard seeds pop, add the steamed balls and the grated coconut. Mix well, remove from the heat and serve.

Note

- You can use finger millet flour instead of buckwheat flour in this recipe.

27. Steamed Millet Flour

An easy and healthy steamed breakfast recipe

Makes: 3 cups; Preparation time: 10 minutes; Resting time: 15–20 minutes; Cooking time: 15 minutes; Effect on doshas: K-

Ingredients

- ¼ cup water
- ¼ tsp rock salt

- 1 cup pearl millet flour
- ¼ cup coconut, grated
- 2 tsp ghee

Method

- Heat water in a saucepan. When the water becomes hot (not boiling), add the salt and mix well.
- Add this water little by little to the pearl millet flour and mix thoroughly. Make sure there are no lumps. It should not become a paste or be too dry. Now cover with a lid and leave it for 15–20 minutes.
- Now heat an idli steamer and spread this wet pearl millet flour in the idli moulds and sprinkle with grated coconut. Cover with a lid and steam for 15 minutes until it is well cooked. Then transfer it to a plate, drizzle ghee over it and serve.

28. Mixed Veg Barley Flatbread

A great power-packed digestive aid

Makes: 6; Preparation time: 30 minutes; Effect on doshas: K-

Ingredients

- 1 tsp fenugreek seeds
- 1¼ cups barley flour + more for dusting
- 1 tsp cumin seeds
- ¼ cup spring onions, finely chopped
- ¼ cup capsicum, finely chopped
- ¼ tsp rock salt, or as per taste
- 2 tsp coriander leaves, finely chopped
- ½–¾ cup water
- 4–5 tsp ghee

Method

- Soak the fenugreek seeds in water overnight. The next morning, discard the water.
- In a bowl, add the barley flour, fenugreek seeds, cumin seeds, spring onions, capsicum, salt and coriander leaves and mix well.
- Now add the water to this mixture in parts and knead to make a uniform dough. Cover with a wet cloth or a lid and leave it for 15–20 minutes.
- Then divide the dough into lemon-sized portions. Take 1 portion and dust it lightly with barley flour. Using a rolling pin, roll it out on the rolling platform into an even disc, about ¼ inch thick and 4 inches in diameter. Make sure it is rolled evenly and is not too thick or too thin.
- Heat a griddle and transfer the disc on to it. When the base has brown spots, flip it to cook the other side.
- Remove from the griddle, drizzle ghee over it and serve hot with yoghurt or vegetables.
- Repeat with the remaining dough.

29. Spinach Flatbread

A perfect meal with a low glycaemic index that keeps your hunger pangs away

Makes: 5; Preparation time: 10 minutes; Resting time: 20 minutes; Cooking time: 25 minutes; Effect on doshas: P- K- V+

Ingredients

- ¼ cup spinach leaves, chopped
- ¼ cup + 3–4 tsp water
- 1¼ cups pearl millet flour
- ¼ tsp ginger, grated
- ½ tsp black pepper, crushed

- ½ tsp cumin powder
- ½ tsp turmeric powder
- ½ tsp sesame seeds
- ¼ tsp rock salt, or as per taste
- 6 tsp sesame oil (divided into 1 tsp + 5 tsp)

Method

- In a pan, add the spinach leaves and 3–4 tsp water, cover with a lid and cook on a low flame for about 2–3 minutes or until the spinach leaves are cooked. Remove the leaves from the heat and let them cool to room temperature. Then blend the leaves into a fine paste along with the water, using a hand blender or mixer-grinder.
- In a bowl, add the pearl millet flour, the spinach paste, ginger, black pepper, cumin, turmeric, sesame seeds, salt, the remaining water and 1 tsp oil. Mix well using a spatula or knead well to make a soft dough. If required (that is, if the mixture is too dry), you may add a little water to make the dough. Cover the dough with a lid or a wet cloth and leave it for about 20 minutes.
- Then divide the dough into golf-ball-sized portions.
- Take 1 ball and flatten it using your palm to make a disc of moderate thickness. Then sprinkle some pearl millet flour on both sides.
- Heat a skillet on medium-high heat. While the skillet is getting hot, start flattening the dough ball further using your palms or place the dough ball between 2 sheets of parchment paper and press using your hands or a bowl with a flat base, to make a flat round disc of even thickness. The disc may crack or break if you try to flatten it using a rolling platform and pin because of the lack of gluten in the flour. Once the disc is prepared, gently place it on the hot skillet and maintain moderate heat.
- In 2–3 minutes, you will see small bubbles appearing on the surface. This means the other side is half-cooked. Now apply sesame oil to grease the surface and flip the disc using a spatula to cook the other side.

- The flatbread will puff up. Now apply sesame oil on this side too and press on the centre and the edges gently. Cook until golden to dark brown spots appear on the surface. Then remove from the skillet and place it on a plate.
- Repeat with the rest of the dough and keep stacking them on a plate. Serve hot with yoghurt or a spread.

30. Maize Flatbread

A comforting gluten-free recipe packed with macro- and micro-nutrients to keep you warm this winter

Makes: 7; Preparation time: 10 minutes; Resting time: 20 minutes; Cooking time: 30 minutes; Effect on doshas: K-

Ingredients

- 2 cups maize flour + more for dusting
- 1 tsp bishop's weed
- ¼ tsp rock salt, or as per taste
- ½ tsp turmeric powder
- ¾ cup warm water
- 7–8 tsp sesame oil

Method

- In a bowl, add the maize flour, bishop's weed, rock salt and turmeric powder and mix using a spatula. Now add the warm water in parts while kneading the mixture by hand or mixing it with a spatula.
- After kneading for 3–5 minutes, the dough will become smooth and firm. You can adjust the water based on the texture of the dough. It should not be too dry or too sticky. The dough should not stick to the sides of the bowl or your hands. If it is sticking, you may grease your hands with ½ tsp sesame oil and knead the dough till it is smooth. Cover with a lid or a wet cloth and leave it for 20 minutes.

- Make golf-ball-sized balls of dough.
- Heat a skillet on medium-high heat. Meanwhile take 1 ball, dust it with a little maize flour and place it on a rolling platform.
- Grease your palm with oil and flatten the ball gently to get a round disc with moderate thickness. Alternatively, you may place a parchment paper or polythene sheet over the dough ball and press it with your hands or a bowl with a flat base to make a flat round disc of even thickness.
- Now cook the discs in the same way as mentioned in the Mixed Veg Barley Flatbread recipe on Pg. 217. Serve with a vegetable or lentil curry.

31. Barley–Millet Fried Bread

A nutritious recipe that helps reduce the risk of metabolic problems and chronic health concerns

Makes: 8; Preparation time: 15 minutes; Resting time: 15–20 minutes; Cooking time: 20–25 minutes; Effect on doshas: K-

Ingredients

- 1 medium-sized potato
- 1¼ cups water (divided into 1 cup + ¼ cup)
- 4 tsp green peas
- 1 cup pearl millet flour
- ½ cup barley flour + more for dusting
- 1 tsp cumin seeds
- 2 pinches bishop's weed
- 1½ tsp sesame seeds
- ½ tsp turmeric powder
- ¼ tsp rock salt, or as per taste
- 2 tsp capsicum, finely chopped

- ¼ cup coriander leaves, finely chopped
- 1 tsp dried fenugreek leaves
- 9 tsp sesame oil (divided into 1 tsp + 8 tsp)

Method

- Wash the potato and cook it with 1 cup of water in a pressure cooker for 2 whistles. Let the pressure go off. Now discard the water and remove the potato from the cooker and peel it.
- In a saucepan, add the green peas and water. Cover with a lid and cook for about 5–7 minutes, until the green peas become soft. Strain and keep the liquid separately.
- Mash the potato and green peas together in a bowl using a masher or a ladle. Keep aside.
- In a bowl, add the pearl millet and barley flours, and mix well. Now add the cumin seeds, bishop's weed, sesame seeds, turmeric powder, salt, capsicum, coriander leaves and dried fenugreek leaves. Mix well.
- Now add the mashed potato-peas mix. And then add the water strained after cooking the peas little by little to the mixture in the bowl while simultaneously kneading it. You will need only a little water so do not add all of it at once. When it becomes a soft dough, grease your palms with 1 tsp of oil and knead once again to remove any flour that is stuck to your hands. Now cover the dough with a wet cloth or a lid and keep it aside for 15–20 minutes.
- Divide the dough into 8 parts. Shape them into balls using your hands. Dust each ball with a little barley flour and roll it out with a rolling pin and board to get a circular disc, about ¼ inch thick. It is not possible to roll out a very thin disc, but if the disc is too thick, it will not cook well and will be difficult to digest. Prepare similar discs from the remaining dough balls.
- Then heat the oil in a deep pan or kadai on medium heat, and when the oil is hot, carefully slide the rolled piece into the oil. When it rises to the surface, gently press it down using a perforated ladle. It will puff up well. Then flip it carefully and fry the other side as well

for 1–2 minutes. This fried lentil bread will be light to dark golden in colour when fried properly. Remove it from the oil and place it in a steel colander so that the excess oil is drained out. Lower the flame and fry the rest of the discs. For more details about the procedure, refer to the Golden Crisp recipe on Pg. 103.
- Serve it hot with a vegetable or lentil curry.

Note
- The dough should not be pasty or too dry. If pasty, add more flour and if dry, add a little more water.

32. Mung Salad

A low-fat and high-protein salad to keep your body weight in check

Makes: 1 cup; Preparation time: 10 minutes; Effect on doshas: K-

Ingredients
- ½ cup spring onions, finely chopped
- 2 garlic cloves, skin peeled, finely chopped
- ½ cup tomatoes, finely chopped
- ¼ cup sprouted mung
- ¼ tsp black pepper powder
- ¼ tsp mustard seed powder
- ¼ tsp rock salt, or as per taste
- 1 tsp olive oil
- 2 tsp coriander leaves, finely chopped
- 2 tsp mint leaves, finely chopped

Method
- In a bowl, add all the ingredients, toss well and serve.

Notes

- You can use sprouted chickpeas instead of sprouted mung in this recipe.
- If you have slow digestion, it will be good to steam the sprouted mung/chickpeas before cooking.
- You can also add ¼ cup of pomegranate to this salad.

33. Millet–Rice Cake

A tasty and nutritious low-carb alternative to the popular south Indian breakfast dish idli, which is usually made with parboiled rice and black lentils

Servings: 18; Soaking time: Overnight; Preparation time: 25 minutes; Fermentation time: Overnight; Cooking time: 25 minutes; Effect on doshas: K- V-

Ingredients

- 1¼ cups foxtail millet
- ½ cup rice, parboiled
- ½ cup whole black lentils, de-husked
- 2 tsp fenugreek seeds
- ¼ cup flattened rice
- 1–1¼ cups water
- ¼ tsp rock salt, or as per taste
- Ghee or sesame oil for greasing

Method

- Wash and soak the foxtail millet and rice together in water overnight. Then discard the water. Wash and soak the black lentils and fenugreek seeds combined in water overnight and then discard the water. Soak the flattened rice in water for 30 minutes and then drain the water using a colander.

- In a mixer-grinder, grind the foxtail millet, the parboiled rice and the flattened rice together using ½ cup of water to a fine granular consistency.
- Grind the lentil and fenugreek together with ¼–½ cup of water to get a smooth, fluffy batter. You can also grind them in batches. If you're grinding in batches, add the water in portions. Make sure not to add too much water as the batter will then attain a watery consistency. The batter should have a thick and flowing consistency.
- In a bowl that has more height than width, add both the batters and salt, mix well and cover with a lid. Leave this batter overnight during winter and for 5–6 hours in the summer to ferment.
- Prepare the cooking equipment (idli steamer or Instant Pot or pressure cooker) in which you are going to place the idli stand. Add 1–2 cups of water to the equipment based on its capacity (the level of water should be just below the first mould of the idli stand) and let the water boil. Now grease the idli moulds using ghee or sesame oil and pour 2 tsp of the batter into each mould. Place the idli stand inside the equipment and cover with a lid that has a steam vent. If you're using a pressure cooker, remove its whistle and place the lid tightly on the cooker. Cook for 12–15 minutes on a moderate flame. You can use the steam option in the Instant Pot to cook it for the same amount of time. Let the idlis sit in the cooking equipment for 5 minutes. Open the lid and remove the idlis using a spoon. Serve hot with chutney or a lentil curry.

Notes

- You can refrigerate the batter for 2–3 days.
- You can also make crepes with this batter.

34. Bean Salad

An easy and nutrient-dense recipe that you'll love

Makes: 1½ cups; Soaking time: Overnight; Preparation time: 25 minutes; Effect on doshas: K-

Ingredients

- ¼ cup kidney beans
- 2–2½ cups water
- ¼ cup corn kernels
- ¼ cup parsley, finely chopped
- ¼ cup carrots, grated
- ½ tsp fresh ginger, grated
- ½ tsp carom seeds
- ½ tsp cumin powder
- 2 seedless dates, finely chopped
- 1 tsp lemon juice
- 1 tsp capers, chopped

Method

- Soak the kidney beans in water overnight. Then discard the water.
- Heat 2 cups of water in a pan, add the soaked kidney beans and cook on a moderate flame. After 20 minutes, add the corn kernels and keep cooking for 5 minutes. Then remove the pan from the heat, strain and transfer the kidney beans and corn to a bowl. Add chopped parsley, grated carrots, ginger, carom seeds, cumin powder, dates, lemon juice and capers, mix well and serve.

Notes

- You can prepare this recipe using white beans instead of kidney beans.
- You can use marjoram or oregano instead of carom seeds and pickled green peppers instead of capers.

35. Fenugreek Chaat

A superfood that burns fat and improves overall health

Makes: 2 cups; Preparation time: 10 minutes; Effect on doshas: K-

Ingredients

- 1 cup sprouted fenugreek seeds (for details about how to make sprouts, see Pgs. 63–65)
- ¼ cup cucumber, chopped
- ¼ cup spring onions, chopped
- ¼ cup tomato, chopped
- 2 tsp mint leaves, finely chopped
- 1 tsp ginger, grated
- 1 tsp cumin powder
- 1 tsp black pepper, crushed
- 1 tsp lemon juice

Method

- In a bowl, add all the ingredients, mix well and serve.

Note

- You can replace fenugreek seeds with sprouted finger millet.

36. Broccoli–Peas Soup

This vibrant, flavour-packed green soup is best enjoyed in winter

Makes: 4 cups; Preparation time: 30 minutes; Effect on doshas: K-

Ingredients

- 2 tsp sesame oil

- 1 cup onion, finely chopped
- 1 garlic clove, finely chopped
- 2 cups broccoli, finely chopped (florets and stem separately)
- ¼ tsp fenugreek powder
- 1 cup green peas
- 4 cups water
- ¼ cup basil leaves, finely chopped
- 2 tsp pineapple juice
- ¼ tsp rock salt, or as per taste
- ¾ tsp black pepper powder

Method

- In a thick-bottomed vessel, heat the sesame oil and when it is hot, add the onion and sauté for 4–5 minutes.
- Then add the garlic and broccoli stem and sauté for 2–3 minutes.
- Add the fenugreek powder, broccoli florets and water. Bring to a boil.
- Next, add the green peas and cook for 3–4 minutes until the broccoli is tender.
- Remove from the heat and add the basil leaves and pineapple juice. Blend the mixture using a hand blender.
- Add salt and black pepper. Mix well and serve.

Note

- You can use 1 tsp lemon juice instead of pineapple juice in the recipe.

37. Protein Leek Soup

A zingy soup with a satisfying taste, texture and nutrient profile

Makes: 4 cups; Soaking time: Overnight; Cooking time: 45 minutes; Effect on doshas: K-

Ingredients

- ½ cup white beans
- 2 tsp sesame oil
- 2 leeks, sliced into ¼-inch slices after cutting and discarding the white bulb
- 1 cup kale, finely chopped
- 3 cups water
- Rock salt as per taste
- ½ tsp black pepper powder

Method

- Soak the white beans in water overnight. Then discard the water.
- Transfer the soaked white beans to a pressure cooker, add 3 cups of water and cook for 5–6 whistles. Remove from the heat and wait for the pressure to go off. Then filter to separate the beans and the liquid.
- In a large skillet, heat the sesame oil and when it is hot, add the leeks and sauté for 3–5 minutes or until the leeks become soft.
- Now add the kale and sauté for another 3–5 minutes. Then add the liquid from the cooked beans. Cook over a medium flame for 20–25 minutes.
- Now add the beans and cook for another 5 minutes. Then remove from the heat, add the salt and black pepper and serve hot.

Note

- You can also puree the mixture using a hand blender before adding the beans and condiments.

38. Amaranth Veggie Mix

A hearty, satisfying and incredibly tasty meal best consumed during autumn or winter

Makes: 2 cups; Soaking time: Overnight; Preparation time: 30 minutes; Effect on doshas: K-

Ingredients

- ½ cup grain amaranth
- 4 garlic cloves, finely chopped
- ½-inch piece fresh ginger, peeled, finely chopped
- ¾ cup water
- ¼ tsp salt, or as per taste
- 10–12 almonds, finely chopped
- 1 dry fig, finely chopped
- ½-inch piece cinnamon
- 2 cloves
- ½ tsp dill seeds
- ¾ tsp fenugreek seeds
- 2 tsp sesame oil
- ¾ cup vegetables (broccoli, cauliflower, cabbage, beets, brussels sprouts, mushrooms, onions, bell peppers), chopped into ½-inch pieces
- 2 tsp corn kernels
- 1 tsp green peas
- 4–5 whole black peppercorns, crushed
- 4–5 basil leaves, finely chopped
- 4–5 mint leaves, finely chopped
- 4–5 cherry tomatoes, chopped into halves

Method

- Wash and soak the grain in water overnight. Then drain the water.
- In a pressure cooker or thick-bottomed vessel, add the grain along with the garlic, fresh ginger, water and salt and cook for 3 whistles

- in the pressure cooker or for about 35 minutes in the open vessel. If using an open vessel, you may have to add an additional ¼ cup of water.
- In a shallow frying pan, dry roast the nuts and dry fruits on medium heat until they emit a nice aroma. Transfer them to a plate. In the same pan, dry roast the cinnamon, cloves, dill seeds and fenugreek seeds for 1–2 minutes. Transfer to the same plate.
- Now smear the pan with 2 tsp oil and increase the heat to medium-high. Add the chopped vegetables, corn kernels and green peas and roast them until they turn brown, that is, about 7–10 minutes. Make sure not to burn them. You may stir them a few times but not too much. When the vegetables are roasted, add the crushed black pepper, mix well and transfer the vegetables to a large bowl. Then add the cooked grain to it and garnish with the basil and mint leaves, cherry tomatoes, roasted nuts and dry fruits along with the roasted spices. Serve.

Notes

- If your pan is small, you can roast the vegetables in small batches. Spread the vegetables evenly on the pan while roasting them. There should be space between the vegetables and no overlapping so that they get roasted evenly. Every time you roast a new batch, smear the pan with a little oil beforehand.
- You can use other wholegrains like rye, barley or millets instead of amaranth.

39. Buckwheat Veggie Crunch

This recipe combines mixed vegetables and buckwheat groats to make a simple meal packed with nutrients.

Makes: 3 cups; Preparation time: 25–30 minutes; Effect on doshas: K-

Ingredients

- 2 tsp sesame oil (divided into 1 tsp + 1 tsp)
- 1 cup buckwheat groats
- ½ tsp mustard seeds
- ¼ tsp cumin seeds
- 5–6 curry leaves
- ¾ tsp fresh ginger, grated
- ½ cup vegetables (onion, cabbage, beans), finely chopped
- 6 tsp green peas
- 2 cups water
- ½ tsp rock salt, or as per taste

Method

- Heat a skillet, add 1 tsp sesame oil and when it is hot, add the buckwheat groats and fry on a low flame for 7–10 minutes, while stirring occasionally, until it turns lightly aromatic. Transfer to a plate.
- In the same skillet, heat 1 tsp sesame oil. Now add the mustard seeds and when they splutter, add the cumin and the curry leaves and sauté for a minute.
- Then add fresh ginger, chopped vegetables and peas and sauté for 2–3 minutes.
- Now add the buckwheat and the salt.
- Meanwhile, heat the water in a saucepan and add it slowly to the mix of vegetables and buckwheat and mix well. Make sure there are no lumps. Let it cook on a low flame for 15–20 minutes or until the buckwheat is well-cooked. Stir occasionally to prevent the mixture from sticking to the bottom. Serve.

Notes

- Other vegetables like carrots, cauliflower or broccoli can also be used instead of the vegetables mentioned in the recipe.

- You can also use semolina, oats or cracked wheat instead of buckwheat groats. The use of semolina or cracked wheat helps reduce Vata dosha.

40. Millet Kitchari

A healthy and well-balanced nutritional punch especially for the spring

Makes: ¾ cup; Soaking time: Overnight; Cooking time: 15–20 minutes; Effect on doshas: K-

Ingredients

- ¼ cup Kodo millet or little millet
- 4 tsp brown lentils
- 1 cup water
- 1 tsp ghee
- ½ tsp black peppercorns
- ½ tsp cumin seeds
- 2 pinches asafoetida
- 5–6 curry leaves
- 1 tsp capsicum, finely chopped
- ½ tsp fresh ginger, grated
- ¼ tsp turmeric powder
- ¼ tsp rock salt, or as per taste
- 1 tsp coriander leaves, finely chopped

Method

- Wash and soak the Kodo or little millet and brown lentils in 1 cup of water overnight. Next morning drain the water and discard it.
- Heat a pressure cooker on a moderate flame. Add ghee and when it is hot, add the black peppercorns, cumin seeds, asafoetida and sauté for half a minute.

- Now add curry leaves, capsicum, ginger, turmeric powder and sauté for another half a minute.
- After that, add the millet and the brown lentils. Fry for a minute.
- Then add 1 cup of water and salt. Mix well and when it comes to a boil, cover with the lid and cook for 4 whistles on a medium flame.
- Let the pressure release by itself. Now open the lid and mix well. Garnish with coriander leaves and serve hot with a lentil curry.

41. Seasoned Yoghurt

A probiotic and protein-rich, easy-to-prepare, aromatic lentil–yoghurt recipe that is very helpful for digestion and gut health and for calibrating metabolic functions.

Makes: 4 cups; Soaking time: 30 minutes; Preparation time: 20 minutes; Cooking time: 25 minutes; Effect on doshas: K- V- P+

Ingredients

- ¼ cup pigeon peas
- 1½ cups low-fat yoghurt
- ½ tsp black pepper powder
- ¼ tsp rock salt, or as per taste
- 3 cups water (divided into 1 cup + 2 cups)
- 1 tsp mustard/sesame oil
- 2 pinches asafoetida
- ½ tsp turmeric powder

Method

- Wash and soak the pigeon peas in water for 30 minutes. Then discard the water.

- Cook the pigeon peas with 1 cup of water in a pressure cooker on a medium flame for 3–4 whistles. When the pressure goes off, remove the lid of the cooker and allow the pigeon peas to cool down to room temperature.
- Now add the yoghurt, black pepper powder, salt and water to it. Blend it using a hand blender.
- In a pan, add the oil and when it is hot, add the asafoetida and turmeric. Then add the blended pigeon peas–yoghurt mixture slowly and cook it on a medium flame. Keep stirring in between so that it does not stick to the bottom.
- The mixture will start to boil in about 15 minutes. Then lower the heat and simmer for 6–7 minutes. The mixture will thicken. If you prefer it to be thinner, you may add a cup of hot water and mix well. Remove from the heat and serve with rice or flatbreads.

Notes

- If you're cooking the pigeon peas in an open vessel, add 2 cups of water to it and cook for about 20–25 minutes on a moderate flame, till they are cooked to a soft texture.
- You can add finely chopped vegetables while cooking the yoghurt. The vegetables that can be used are onions, tomatoes, carrots, green peas, garlic and ginger. The vegetables should be added after the asafoetida and turmeric, and sautéed for 5–7 minutes. Then add the blended pigeon peas–yoghurt mixture and cook as mentioned in the method section.

42. Spinach Yoghurt

With simple ingredients, this ultra-flavourful, creamy and versatile recipe can be prepared quickly.

Makes: 1 cup; Preparation time: 10 minutes; Effect on doshas: K-

Ingredients

- ¼ cup spinach, finely chopped
- 2 tsp water
- 1 cup low-fat yoghurt
- ½ tsp sesame oil
- ¼ tsp mustard seeds
- ¼ tsp black pepper, crushed
- ½ tsp roasted cumin seeds, crushed
- ¼ tsp rock salt, or as per taste

Method

- Combine the finely chopped spinach and water in a saucepan, cover with a lid and cook on a low flame for 2–3 minutes. Then remove the pan from the heat and when the spinach cools down to room temperature, transfer it to a bowl.
- Add the yoghurt to it, whisk it and keep it aside.
- In another pan, heat the sesame oil and when it is hot, add the mustard seeds. When they splutter, transfer them to the spinach–yoghurt mix.
- Add the salt, black pepper and cumin seeds, mix well and serve.

Note

- You can replace black pepper with grated fresh ginger.

43. Yam Smash

A delicious relish that reduces inflammation and boosts immunity, this recipe is especially good for women going through menopause.

Makes: 3 cups; Preparation time: 30 minutes; Effect on doshas: V- K-

Ingredients

- 3 medium-sized yams, whole
- 2¼ cups water (divided into 2 cups + ¼ cup)
- ½ tsp tamarind paste
- Rock salt as per taste
- ½ tsp turmeric powder
- 2 tsp sesame oil
- ½ cup onion, minced
- 3 garlic cloves, minced

Method

- Add the yams and 2 cups of water to a pressure cooker and cook them for up to 3 whistles.
- When the pressure goes off, pierce the yams with a fork to see if they are cooked. If they are not tender/well cooked, then boil them on a moderate flame for 5–7 minutes more without the lid. Now drain the water and allow the yams to cool down to room temperature. Then peel off the skin of the yams and smash them using a potato masher.
- Add the tamarind paste, salt and turmeric powder to the mashed yams and mix well.
- Heat a skillet and add the sesame oil. When the oil is hot, add the minced onion and garlic, sauté for 4–5 minutes or until the onions turn transparent.
- Then add the smashed yam and sauté for 5 minutes.
- Now add ¼ cup water, mix well and cook on a low flame for 7–10 minutes while stirring occasionally.
- The mixture will thicken and will not stick to the bottom of the skillet. Remove from the heat and serve with rice or flatbreads.

Note

- Tamarind paste can be replaced with 1 tsp lemon juice. If you're using lemon juice, it should be added at the end, after removing the mixture from the heat.

44. Veg Stir-Fry

This is a delicious and quick side dish that preserves nutrients, aids in healthy weight management and is easily customizable.

Makes: 1 cup; Preparation time: 25 minutes; Effect on doshas: V- K-

Ingredients

- 1 tsp sesame oil
- ¼ tsp dill seeds
- 2 garlic cloves, crushed or chopped
- 1 tsp fresh ginger, grated
- ½ cup cauliflower, chopped into florets
- ½ cup beans, chopped into ½-inch pieces
- ¼ cup capsicum, seeds removed, diced
- 6 tsp water
- 1 tsp dried fenugreek leaves
- ¼ tsp black pepper, crushed
- 4–5 pinches salt

Method

- Heat a skillet on a moderate to high flame and add 1 tsp of sesame oil. When it is hot, add the dill seeds, garlic, fresh ginger, cauliflower, beans and capsicum and sauté for 2 minutes.
- Now reduce the heat and add the water, cover with a lid and cook for 10–12 minutes while stirring occasionally.

- Then remove the lid and check if the vegetables are soft by piercing the cauliflower with a fork. If it is not well cooked, add 2 more tsp of water, cover and cook for 3–5 minutes. Then add the dried fenugreek leaves, black pepper and salt.
- Remove from the heat and serve with rice or flatbreads.

45. Eggplant Shallow Fry

This nutrient-dense, low-calorie recipe supports heart and digestive health.

Makes: 2 cups; Preparation time: 30 minutes; Effect on doshas: K-

Ingredients
- 5 eggplants (medium size)
- 4 tsp sesame oil
- 1 pinch asafoetida
- ¼ tsp mustard seeds
- ¼ tsp fenugreek seeds
- ¼ tsp fennel seeds
- ¼ tsp cumin seeds
- ¼ tsp nigella seeds
- 1-inch piece cinnamon stick
- ½ tsp black peppercorns
- 1 tsp tamarind paste
- 3 tsp water
- ¼ tsp rock salt, or as per taste
- ¼ tsp turmeric powder
- ½ tsp coriander powder
- ¾ tsp jaggery

Method

- Wash the eggplants. Then wipe them dry with a cloth or paper towel. Now make 4 slits in each eggplant with the stem at the back intact.
- Heat oil in a frying pan and fry all the eggplants on a moderate flame until they attain a golden colour. This should take about 4–5 minutes. You may also fry them in batches if you have a small frying pan. Remove the eggplants and keep them on a plate.
- Now in the same oil, add the asafoetida and the seeds of mustard, fenugreek, fennel, cumin and nigella. When the mustard seeds pop, add the cinnamon stick and peppercorns. Sauté for a minute.
- Then add tamarind paste, water, salt, turmeric powder and coriander powder. Mix well. Cover and cook for 5 minutes.
- Add the jaggery powder and cook for another 2 minutes.
- Finally add the fried eggplants, cover and cook on medium heat for 5–7 minutes until the eggplants are soft. Serve hot with flatbreads or rice.

46. Crunchy Amaranth Stir-Fry

A super simple recipe with a nutty flavour and a spicy kick

Makes: 1 cup; Preparation time: 20 minutes; Effect on doshas: P- K-

Ingredients

- ¼ cup raw peanuts
- 2 cups amaranth leaves, washed, finely chopped
- 2 tsp sesame oil (divided into 1 tsp + 1 tsp)
- 1 tsp cumin seeds
- ½ tsp poppy seeds
- 2 garlic cloves, finely chopped
- ½ tsp ginger, grated

- ½ tsp black pepper, crushed
- ¼ tsp rock salt, or as per taste

Method

- Dry roast the peanuts in a skillet on a moderate flame for about 10 minutes or until they become crispy. Make sure to stir occasionally to prevent the peanuts from getting burnt. Then remove from the heat and let them cool down to room temperature. Crush them coarsely using a hand pounder.
- In the same skillet, heat 1 tsp oil and add the amaranth leaves. Cook on high heat for 2 minutes, then reduce the flame to medium heat and cook until the amaranth leaves become tender. Stir at frequent intervals.
- Heat the remaining oil in another skillet and add the cumin seeds. When they brown, add the poppy seeds, garlic and ginger and sauté for 1–2 minutes. Add the black pepper and remove from the heat. Now add this tempering to the cooked amaranth along with the peanuts.
- Add salt, mix well and serve.

47. Tangy Turnip

An easy, healthy and flavourful turnip curry with bold flavours

Makes: 1½ cups; Preparation time: 20 minutes; Effect on doshas: V- K-

Ingredients

- 1 tsp sesame oil or ghee
- 4–5 pinches asafoetida
- ½ cup shallots, thinly sliced
- 1 cup turnip, skin lightly peeled, diced
- ¼ cup water

- ½ tsp rock salt
- 1 tsp tamarind paste
- 1 tsp cumin powder
- 2 tsp coriander powder
- ½ tsp turmeric powder
- 1½ tsp black pepper powder

Method

- Heat a skillet on a medium flame and add the ghee.
- Add the asafoetida and shallots and sauté for 2 minutes. Then add the diced turnips, water and salt. Cover and cook for 7–10 minutes on a low flame or until the turnips become tender.
- Now add the tamarind paste, cumin, coriander, turmeric and black pepper. Cover and cook for 3–5 minutes more.
- Remove the lid and check if the turnips are well cooked. Make sure not to mash or overcook the turnips. If there is excess water, heat the turnips on a low flame after removing the lid so that it evaporates. Remove from the heat and serve with rice or flatbreads.

48. Peppery Curry

An aromatic, delicious, flavourful gravy that delivers a wonderfully unusual spice hit, this pepper curry is best enjoyed in winter.

Makes: 1 cup; Preparation time: 30 minutes; Effect on doshas: K-

Ingredients

- 2 tsp tamarind paste
- ½ cup water (divided into ¼ cup + ¼ cup)
- 2 tsp coconut oil (divided into 1 tsp + 1 tsp)
- 3 tsp coconut, grated
- 4 tsp coriander seeds

- 1 tsp fennel seeds
- 1 tsp cumin seeds
- 6 tsp black pepper
- 1 tsp fresh ginger, grated
- 5–6 curry leaves
- ½ cup shallots, chopped (divided into ¼ cup + ¼ cup)
- ½ cup garlic, chopped (divided into ¼ cup + ¼ cup)
- 1 tsp ghee

Method

- Dissolve the tamarind paste in ¼ cup water.
- Heat a skillet and add 1 tsp coconut oil. When it is hot, add the coconut, coriander, fennel, cumin, black pepper, fresh ginger, ¼ cup shallots and ¼ cup of garlic and roast them for 4–5 minutes on moderate heat.
- Then transfer the mixture to a plate and let it cool down to room temperature. Grind it to a smooth paste with 2 tsp water in a mixer-grinder. If needed, you can add a little more water.
- Heat another skillet on a moderate flame, add 1 tsp of coconut oil and the curry leaves. Then add the remaining shallots and garlic, and sauté for 3–5 minutes until they are well cooked.
- Then add the tamarind water, the ground mixture and ¼ cup water.
- The mixture will begin to boil. Continue cooking on a moderate flame for 15–20 minutes, until the mixture thickens.
- Remove from the heat, add 1 tsp ghee and serve with rice or idli.

49. Healthy Modak

Being a great source of healthy fats and energy that the body requires to fight off weakness, this is one of the best combinations for taste and health. It is best enjoyed during winter. It is also good for anaemia, amenorrhoea and the postpartum period in a normal delivery.

Makes: 16 balls; Preparation time: 30 minutes; Effect on doshas: K-

Ingredients

- 1 cup ghee
- ¼ cup poppy seeds
- 1 cup sesame seeds
- 6 tsp coconut flakes
- ¼ cup fenugreek powder
- 2½ tsp dry ginger powder
- 2½ tsp black pepper powder
- 2½ tsp long pepper powder
- ¼ cup bishop's weed powder
- 2 cups jaggery powder

Method

- Heat a tawa, add the ghee, then add the poppy seeds and sesame seeds and roast for 12–15 minutes on moderate heat. Next, add the coconut flakes, fenugreek, dry ginger, black pepper, long pepper and bishop's weed powders and sauté for 7–10 minutes.
- Then remove the tawa from the heat and add the jaggery. Mix well and make golf-ball-sized balls of this mixture. Store in a moisture-free airtight container. It stays good for up to 7 days at room temperature and 15 days if refrigerated. Consume 1 ball every day.

50. Millet Bars

A healthy option to satisfy your sugar cravings while trying to lose weight

Makes: 8 bars; Preparation time: 20 minutes; Setting time: 1 hour; Effect on doshas: K-

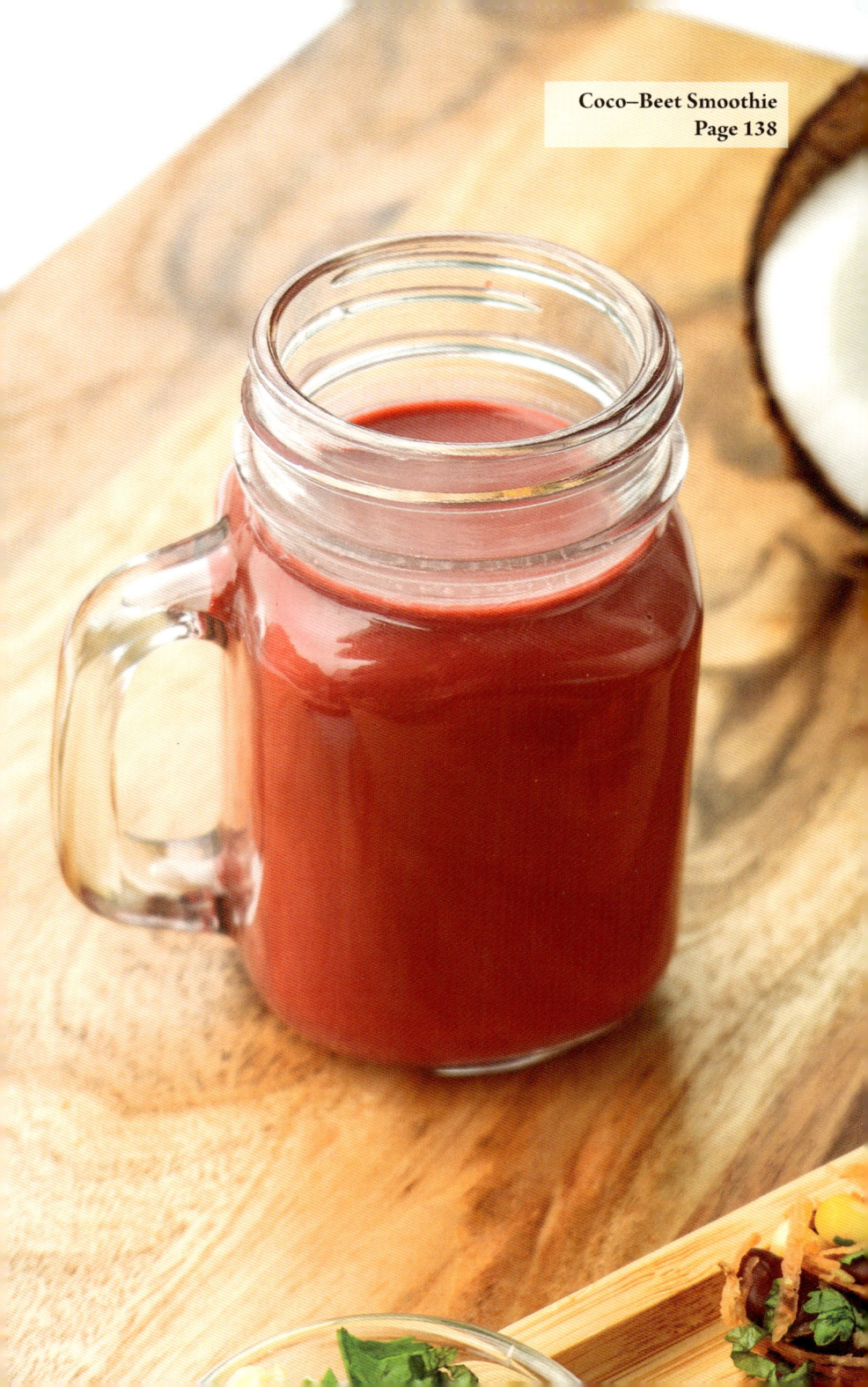

Coco–Beet Smoothie
Page 138

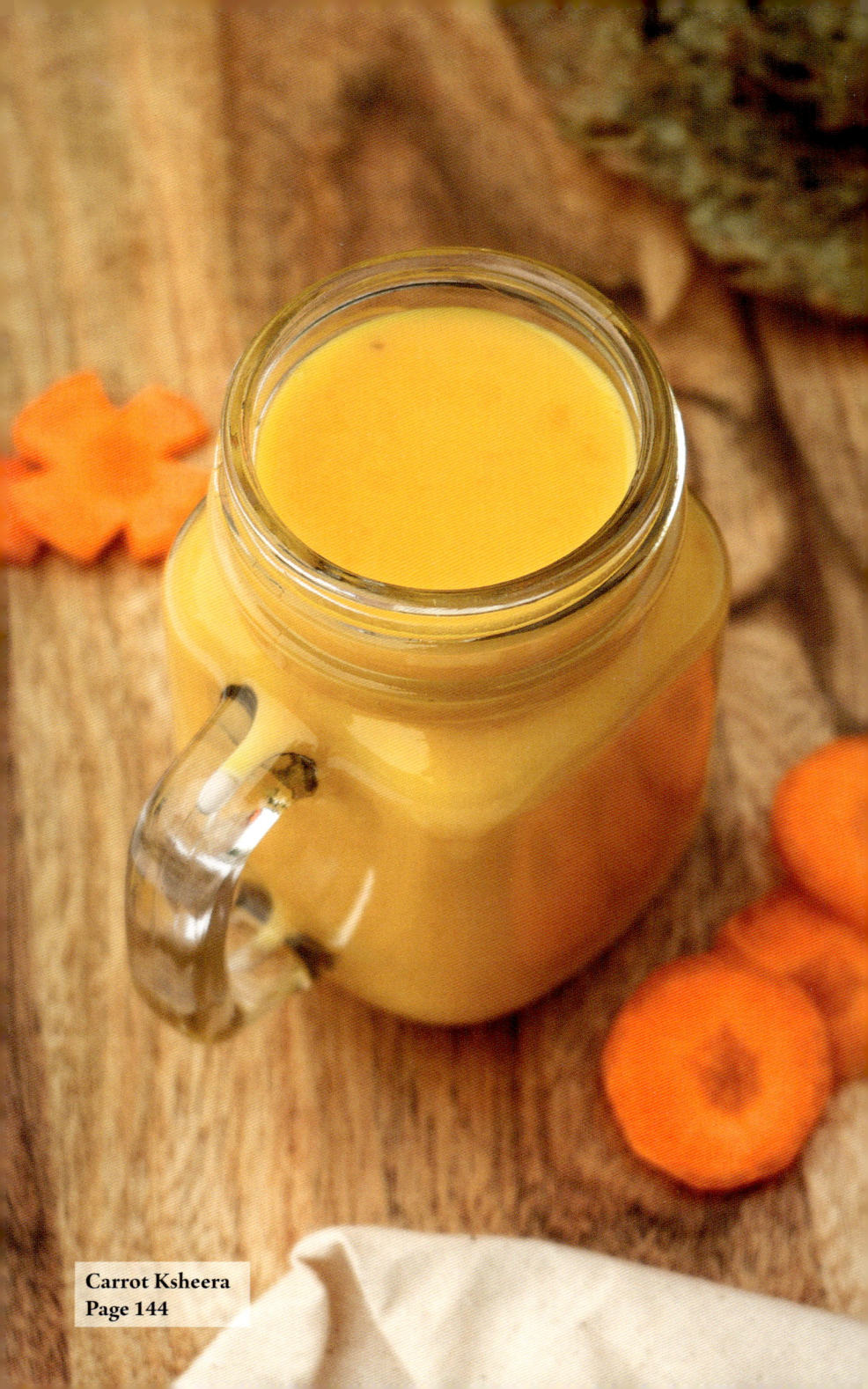

Carrot Ksheera
Page 144

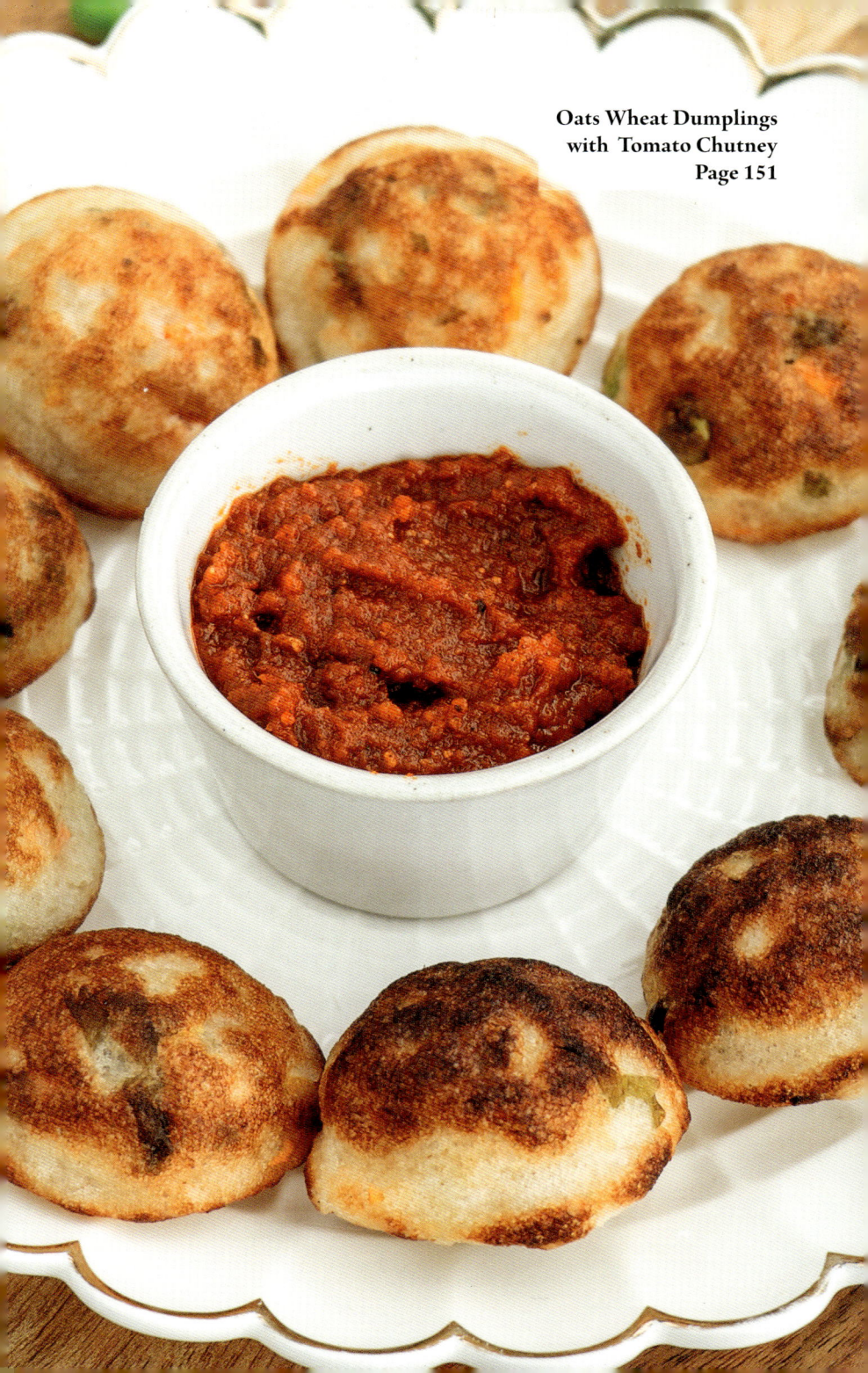

Oats Wheat Dumplings with Tomato Chutney
Page 151

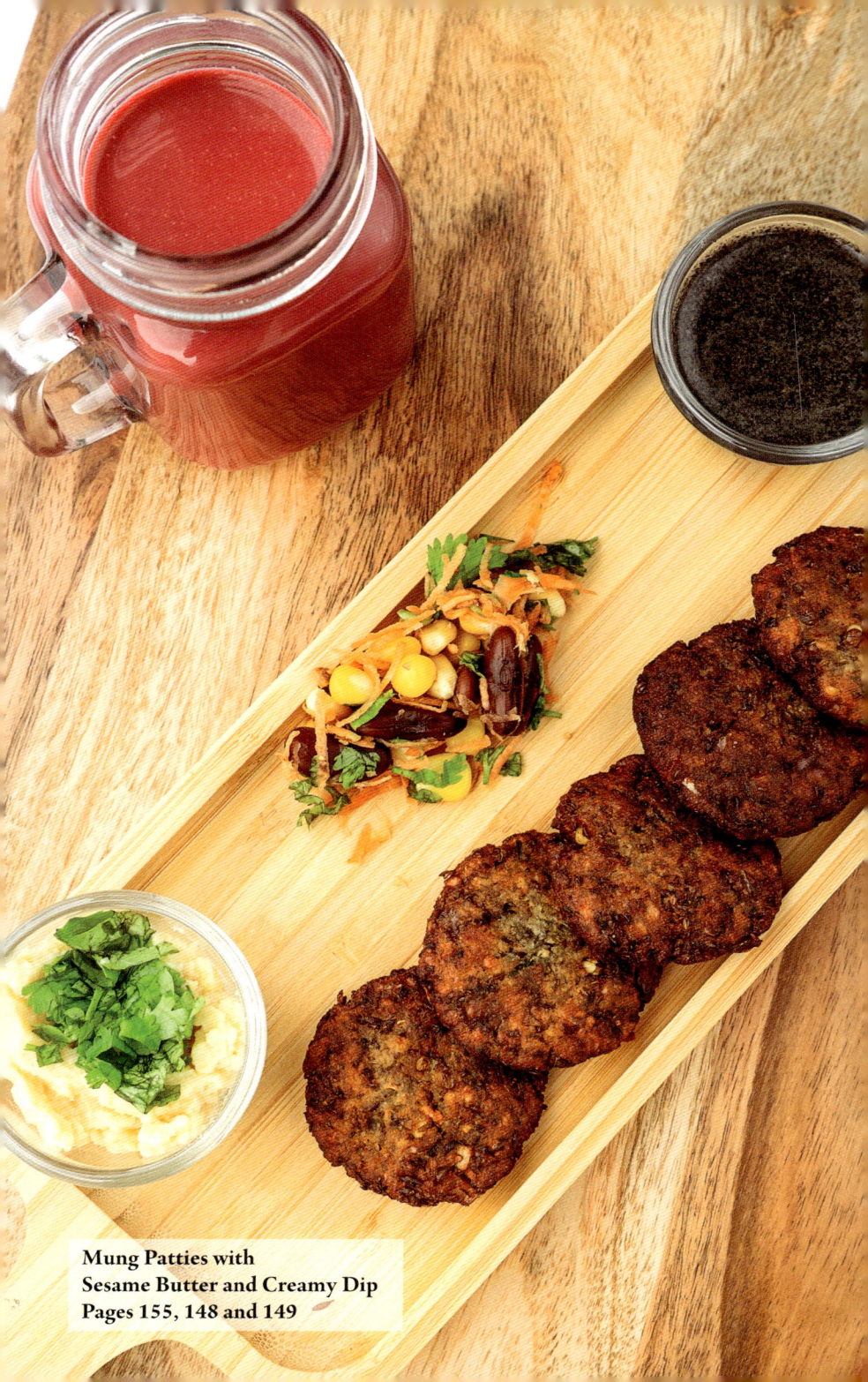

Mung Patties with
Sesame Butter and Creamy Dip
Pages 155, 148 and 149

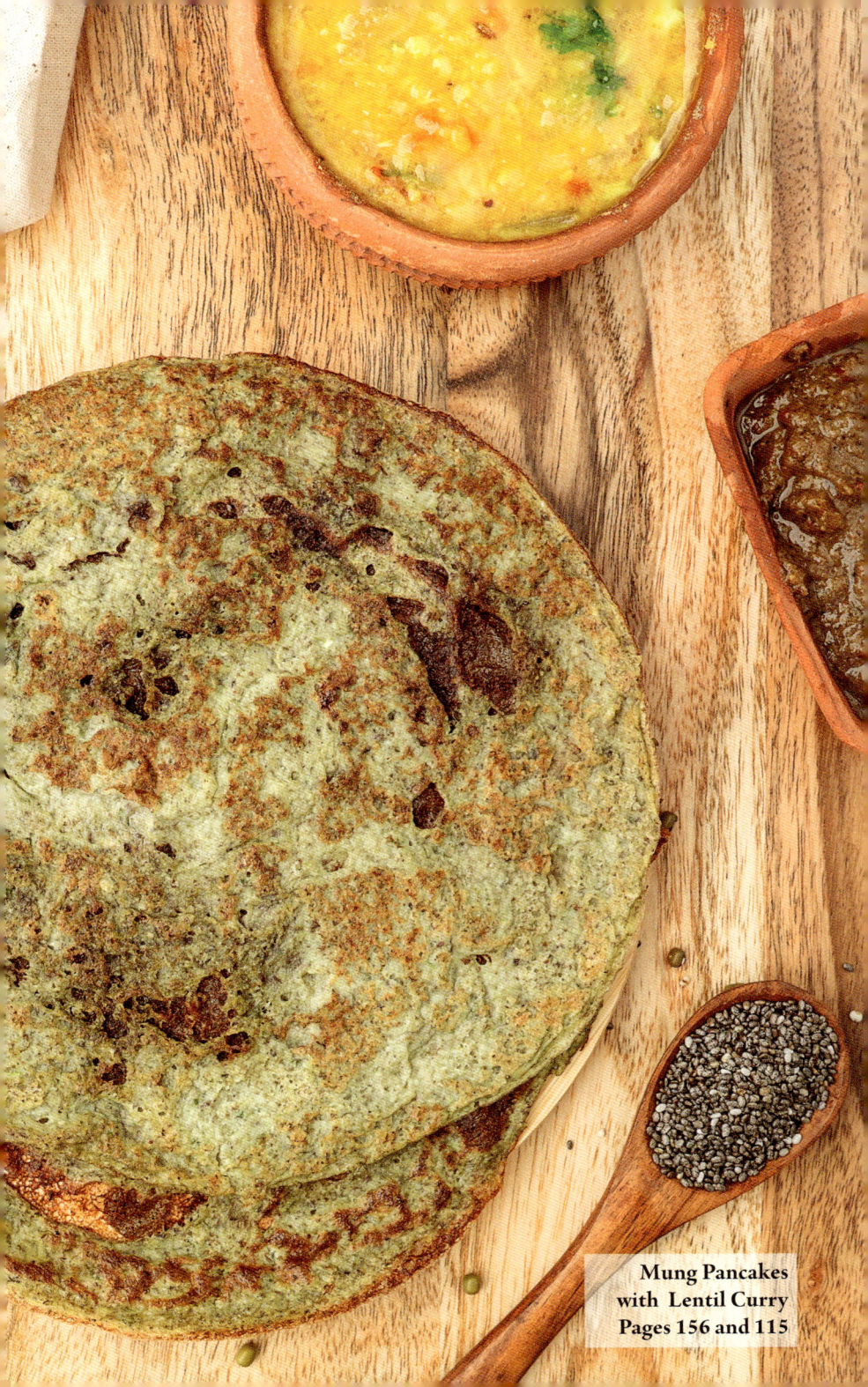

Mung Pancakes with Lentil Curry
Pages 156 and 115

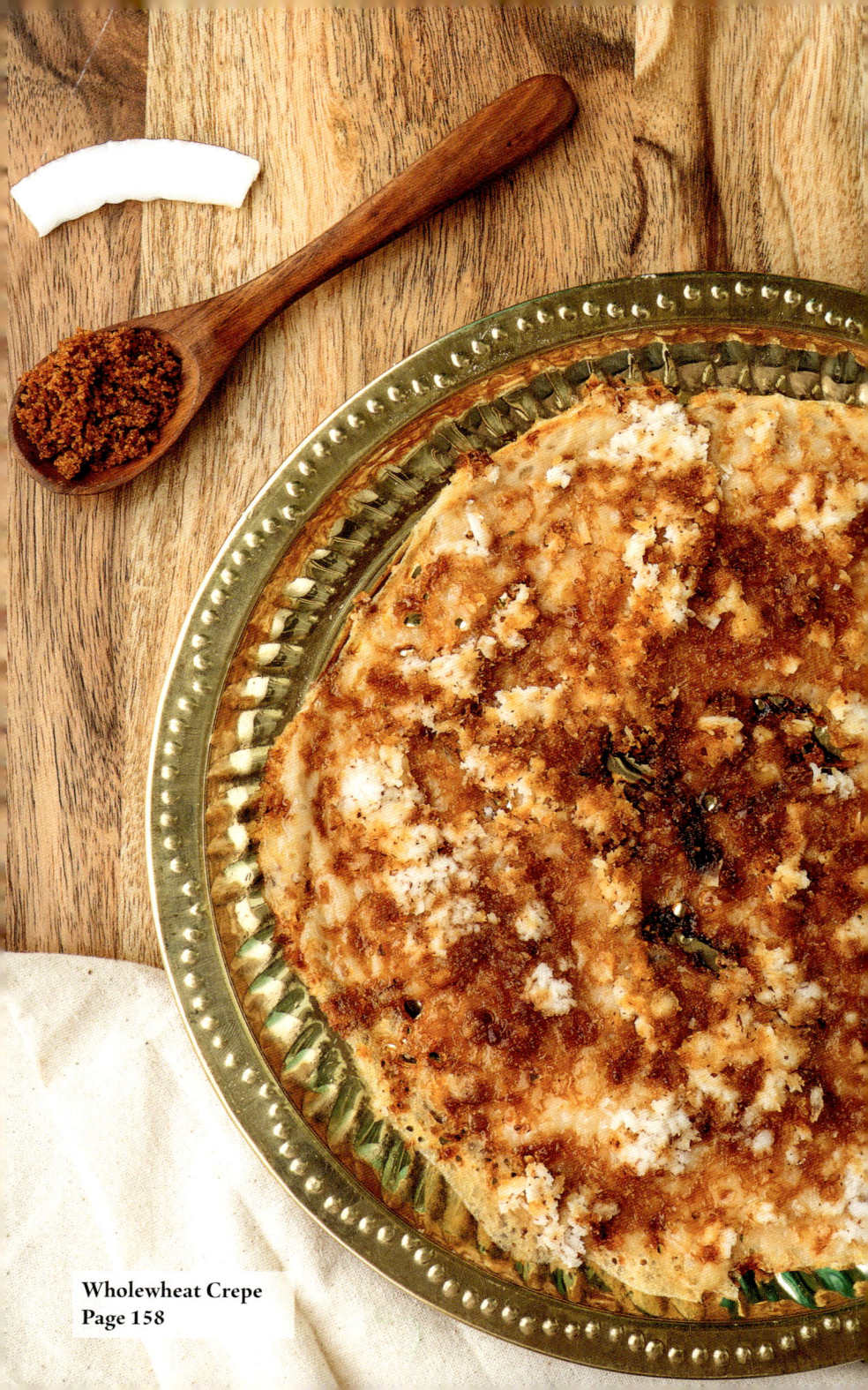

Wholewheat Crepe
Page 158

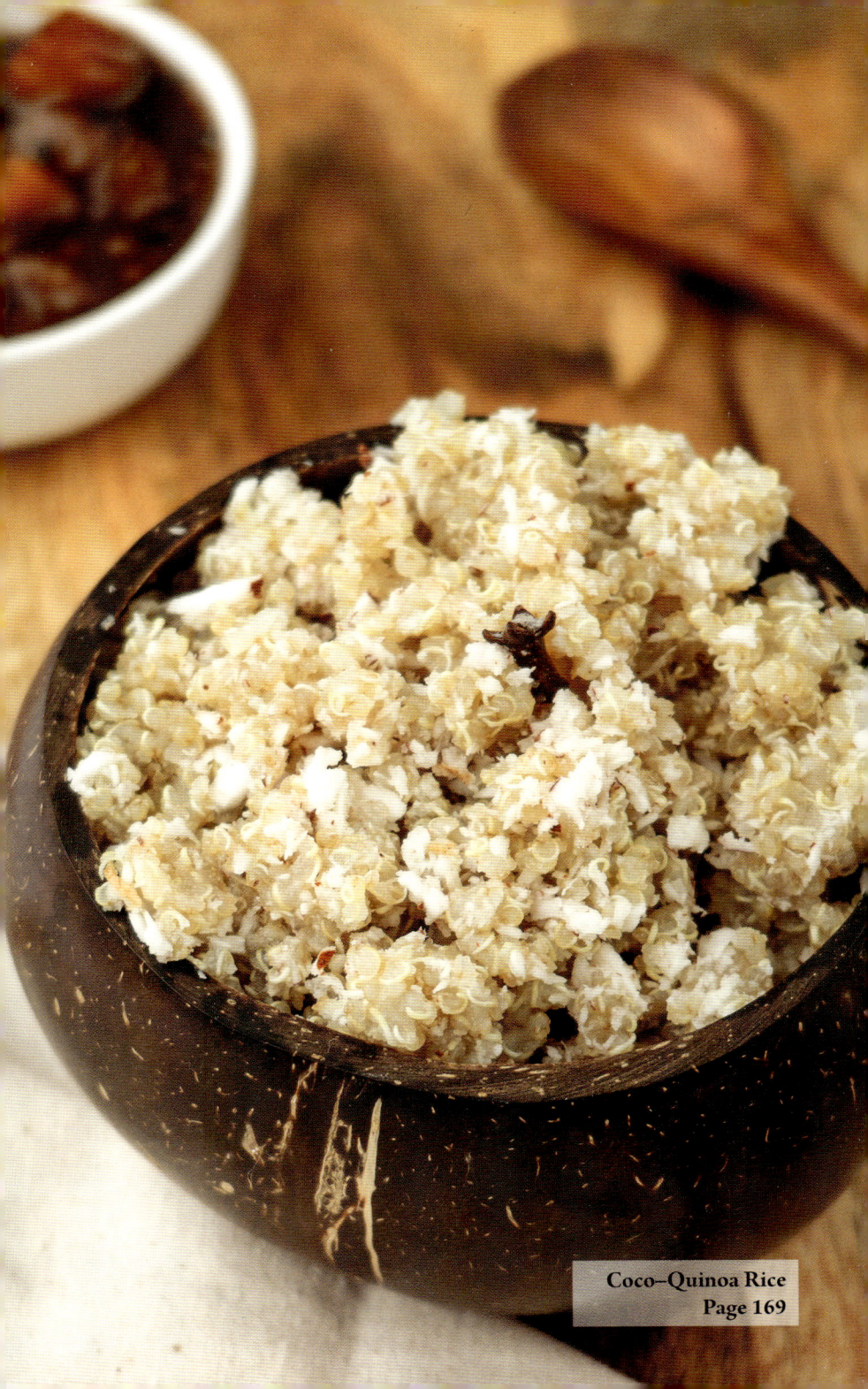

Coco–Quinoa Rice
Page 169

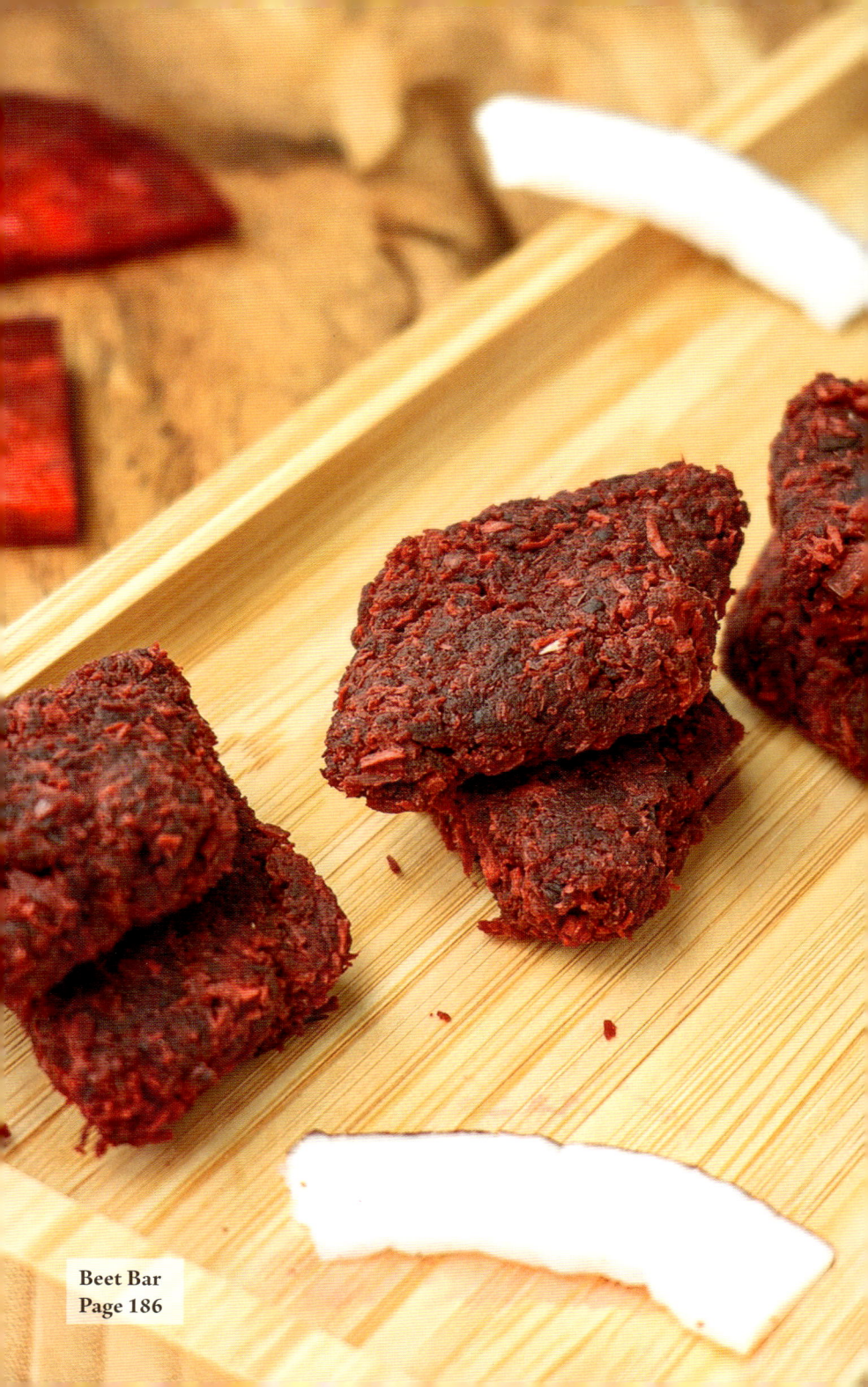

Beet Bar
Page 186

Ingredients

- 1 cup little millet
- 1 tsp flaxseeds
- 2 tsp ghee
- 1 cup jaggery powder
- ½ tsp cardamom powder

Method

- Heat a skillet and dry roast the little millet grains on a moderate flame until they pop. You need to dry roast them in small batches, so you may add ¼ cup to the skillet at a time.
- Transfer the popped millets to a bowl.
- Dry roast the flaxseeds in the same skillet for 1–2 minutes. When they cool down to room temperature, crush the flaxseeds to a coarse powder using a hand pounder.
- Heat 1 tsp of ghee in a pan, add the jaggery powder and sauté for 1–2 minutes, until it becomes a paste.
- Now add the popped millets, flaxseeds and cardamom to the jaggery paste and mix well. Cook it for 1 minute.
- Grease a plate with 1 tsp ghee and transfer the mixture onto it and spread it evenly using a spatula. The layer should be about ½ inch in thickness.
- After 5–7 minutes, when the mixture cools down slightly, cut it into squares using a knife.
- Let them cool down for about 1 hour. Then transfer the pieces to a moisture-free airtight container. Consume 1 bar daily. This stays good for 7 days at room temperature and in the refrigerator for up to 15 days.

ACKNOWLEDGEMENTS

Thanks to the universal spirit for your infinite blessings that helped me channel my energy into writing this book.

I am also grateful for my good health, the love of my family and friends.

I have to start by thanking my wonderful mom. From reading my first drafts to giving me invaluable advice, you were instrumental in the development of this book. Thanks to my dad, who always supported me and never let me down.

A special thanks to my daughter, who provided moments of joy amidst the writing process. Santhini Anoop, I appreciate your patience and understanding during the long hours spent immersed in this book's pursuit.

I am extremely grateful to everyone I've had the chance to lead, be led by, or observe from a distance. You've all inspired me and laid the foundation for this book.

Thanks to my readers for taking the time to read this book.

I would also like to extend my gratitude to Ms Sonavi Kher for her profound belief in my work.

Many thanks to everyone in the publishing team at HarperCollins India for bringing this project to fruition. To my editor, Trisha Bora—I appreciate your insightful suggestions.

Finally, yet importantly, I would like to acknowledge the guidance and wisdom I received from my organization. Thank you, Chakrapani Ayurveda Clinic & Research Center, Jaipur.

NOTES

Scan this QR code to access the notes.

ABOUT THE AUTHOR

Dr Lakshmi Lakshmanan is a passionate physician who teaches holistic living and helps people transform their eating habits to suit their particular body types and health needs. She completed her formal Ayurveda education in Tamil Nadu and worked in south India for a few years. Later, she moved to Jaipur and has been working as a senior physician at the Chakrapani Ayurveda Clinic & Research Center since 2012. She often travels to France and Italy for Ayurveda consultations, conferences and workshops. She has trained many students from all over the world who are now successfully practising as Ayurveda nutritionists, chefs, therapists and wellness counsellors. She has also contributed the topic 'A Traditional Medicine System: Basics of Ayurveda' for the short online course in Integrative Medicine at the National Institute of Integrative Medicine, Australia, in the year 2017.

With over seventeen years of experience, Dr Lakshmi has written about 500 articles on various aspects of holistic living which have been published in different magazines and blogs, including a few review articles and case reports for platforms like the *International Journal of Ayurveda and Pharmaceutical Chemistry*, *Journal of Natural and Ayurvedic Medicine*, *AyuCaRe*, *Global Ayurveda Magazine*, *Ayurveda and All* and *AyurvedSutra*. She has also worked as the editor of the e-newsletter, AyurvedaNews, and the quarterly magazine, *AyurvedaMantra*.

A prolific writer, Dr Lakshmi is the author of *Ayurvedic Prakriti: Who Am I?* She has also edited two other books, *A Beginner's Guide to Ayurveda* and *Vital Points: A Comprehensive Guide to Marma Therapy*.

HarperCollins *Publishers* India

At HarperCollins India, we believe in telling the best stories and finding the widest readership for our books in every format possible. We started publishing in 1992; a great deal has changed since then, but what has remained constant is the passion with which our authors write their books, the love with which readers receive them, and the sheer joy and excitement that we as publishers feel in being a part of the publishing process.

Over the years, we've had the pleasure of publishing some of the finest writing from the subcontinent and around the world, including several award-winning titles and some of the biggest bestsellers in India's publishing history. But nothing has meant more to us than the fact that millions of people have read the books we published, and that somewhere, a book of ours might have made a difference.

As we look to the future, we go back to that one word—a word which has been a driving force for us all these years.

Read.

    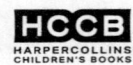

    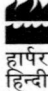